GETTING YOUR EXECUTIVES FIT

GETTING YOUR EXECUTIVES FIT

by
Don T. Jacobs, Ph.D.

Library of Congress Cataloging in Publication Data

Jacobs, Donald T.
    Getting your executives fit.
    Bibliography: p.
    Includes index.
    1. Physical fitness. 2. Exercise. I. Title.
GV341.J25   613.7   79-64731
ISBN 0-89037-176-8

© 1981 by
Donald T. Jacobs

Anderson World, Inc.
Mountain View, California

TABLE OF CONTENTS

To everyone whose potential for living might be stifled by the barriers of civilization to optimal health and fitness.

ACKNOWLEDGMENTS

I would like to thank my wife, Barbara, for her dedicated efforts in typing the final manuscript and for her temporary relinquishing of her own career priorities during the process.

I would also like to express appreciation to Anderson World, Inc. and its staff. Bob Anderson's concern for the wellness of Americans and his courage to challenge the status quo are reflective of the pioneering spirit that will eventually see this book's message to its conclusion.

FOREWORD

The most significant aspect of this work, as I see it, is that it brings the present enthusiasm for health and fitness up to the level of organization and designed social change. It is no news that the power in our society is commanded by organizations—business, political, academic, theological, military, etc. The effectiveness of an individual's creativity may radiate from him/herself as a single entity, or even more out of a diadic relationship, or perhaps out of identification with a family or common-interest group. But it is when that creativity is manifested at the level of organization or institution that it may burst forth to a new, substantially broader scope of effectiveness. A milkman driving his products in from the farm to distribute them to a circle of customers, a privately-owned one-person taxi service, the isolated general practitioner, "country doctor"—these are perhaps delightful nostalgic remembrances of things past, but they are hardly significant effectors in the modern world, which is dominated by their organized institutional counterparts in every sphere.

Organizations, at the same time that they are set up to serve people, tend, by their very natures, to limit individual variation and self-expression. It is simply more efficient to have standardized job and service slots into which real human beings can more or less fit, than to attempt to build or maintain an organization based on individual variation of the people components.

As a result, we come into the modern era which presents us with an incredible technology based on organized, institutionalized labor, goods, management, etc., and which also presents us as individuals with tremendous power and freedom for leisure, self-expression, and varied entertainment. It is an era of extremes of both standardization of individuals and opportunity for individuation.

The great interest in health and fitness of the last decade or two is an outflow of enhancement of the individual. Recently, we have been taught increasingly to cherish our own uniqueness, and nourish our minds and bodies with a sophisticated perspective of self-respect. We have new knowledge, more leisure, and enhanced focus of concern to do this—each of us as an individual.

This book brings a new opportunity and awareness to the level of interaction with organizations. It invites the perspective that this individual enhancement is significant for the health of organizations. It defines for management and its advisers the path toward implementation of this sort of individual enhancement program. It is a neat turn—or return—of evolution that the institutions which so often constrict and routinize us can be turned to organized enhancement of individual experience.

This is perhaps what makes man great and durable; his capacity to create something which is beyond himself, and then regain compassionate control of it to his own enhancement.

—Richard L. Crews, M.D.

INTRODUCTION

The United States is experiencing a revolution. The focus of the revolution is physical fitness. It's not a new theme. Wise men since Plato have tried to impart its virtues to society. But today the need for a fitness revolution is critical, perhaps more critical than ever before. People are more sedentary and are largely unprepared for many social and environmental pressures. Diseases of inactivity are of epidemic proportion. Today's wise men are pleading for people to implement the wisdom of fitness before it is too late.

Unhappily, implementation is not yet significant. In spite of prestigious rhetoric and fitness faddism, little is being done to improve the health of most Americans. Health care costs are creating an economic crisis. Emergency personnel are often in worse condition than the public they are paid to protect. Absenteeism and premature retirement are degrading American productivity. Fitness programs in most schools are inadequate or non-existent. Older persons are wasting the best years of their lives because of unnecessary ill health. The medical community has not been educated to espouse exercise and nutrition priorities seriously.

The problem is that the majority of Americans have not been educated or encouraged to adopt a healthy lifestyle—of which the cornerstone is regular physical activity. Most people do not understand basic nutritional principles or the nature of such vital functions as heart rate or blood pressure. They do not recognize the nature and preventability of the major diseases that plague modern society. They have not been taught the simple guidelines that can make physical fitness and optimal health a pleasant reality. They have not been given opportunities for proper exercise.

If social, economic, and personal health are to exist on a large scale, society must take responsibility for providing opportunities for fitness education and implementation. This book will offer guidelines with which such responsibility can be accepted. It will provide government administrators, employers, employees, educators, parents and concerned citizens with a blueprint for developing efficient and effective fitness programs. Specific guidelines are presented for target populations that comprise or affect the majority of people in the United States. They include business and industry, schools, senior citizens, and communities.

Although guidelines for one group may occasionally be applicable to programs for another, there are motivational, educational, organizational, and implemental needs that are unique to each category. This book's objectives are to:

1. Identify the major obstacles that have impeded health maintenance and fitness programs in the specific grouping.

2. Stimulate an appreciation for the need for fitness programs.

3. Provide organizational guidelines for developing a fitness program.

4. Describe motivational and implemental techniques that will assure an effective and ongoing program.

Special consideration and guidelines for the specific populations will be presented in appropriate chapters. At the outset, however, "Embracing the Basics" will provide the reader with a general understanding of fundamental fitness theory that will augment the political and organizational aspects of fitness program implementation. These theories will be basic to almost every program described herein as well as to most programs endorsed by health and fitness experts throughout the world. These principles are easy to understand and simple to follow and may dispel many misapprehensions about exercise. (For additional information about exercise and nutrition, the bibliography lists several excellent resources.)

Like any movement designed to effect fundamental changes, the fitness "revolution" will meet resistance. In spite of the clear need for improved fitness in many areas, the call for programs may lose momentum. Emerson said that "society is always taken by surprise at any new example of common sense." It is hoped that *Getting Your Executives Fit* will give direction to the fitness movement and will help prepare society to accept an obvious solution without the repercussions of surprise.

PART ONE: EMBRACING THE BASICS

1

A RATIONAL REASON

This book will attest to the fact that there is much to know about organizing fitness programs and motivating people to exercise. Exercise itself is not such a difficult proposition. Until the making of modern civilization nearly everyone was sufficiently active. Civilization, however, has had an unfortunate tendency to de-emphasize physical activity. Attitudes about exercise now exist at opposite extremes that continue to drive each other further apart.

It is a fundamental law of physiology that the functional efficiency of an organ or system improves with use and regresses with disuse. "If you don't use it, you'll lose it." Disuse is the major factor in many bodily changes often thought of as aging. Physical activity is a means of preventing disuse.

The problem is that until recently mankind has not had to think about physical activity. It was an integral part of living. But now that technology and convenience have replaced physical labor and other forms of entertainment have replaced physical recreation, people must begin to think about physical activity in terms of exercise. Exercise is a way of interjecting sufficient doses of physical activity into a modern lifestyle so as to maximize the pleasures and potentialities of life and minimize the atrophy and wasted potential.

This particular view of exercise is worth expanding. By treating exercise as a technological innovation necessary for survival, a less confusing and more practical understanding of exercise can be shared by all. As a person would choose appropriate clothing and equipment for snow skiing, or a proper tool for working, he or she should choose appropriate alternatives for health and well-being. Viewed in this way, exercise would be valued, not in esoteric terms, but in terms of potentiality and functional well-being.

If exercise had been introduced as a more obvious technological innovation, the acceptance of the above view would be widespread. If it existed in the form of a pill, for example, there would be no doubt as to its use. This was reflected in 1705 by Dr. Francis Fuller.

> As for exercise of the body which is the subject of the ensuing discourse, if people would not think so superficially of it, if they would but abstract that benefit got by it from the means by which it is got, they would set a great value on it. If some of the advantages accruing from exercise were to be procured by any one medicine, nothing in the world would be in more esteem than that medicine would be. There is this difference between the most complete productions of human artifice and that fine piece of mechanism—the body of man; that the former are always the worst for wearing and decay by use in motion, the latter, notwithstanding the tenderness of its contexture, improves by exercise and acquires by frequent motion an ability to last the longest.

But exercise is not a pill. It is a task. In spite of the rhetoric preached by many fitness advocates, exercise is not necessarily intrinsically enjoyable. Dr. George Sheehan states that exercise that is not enjoyable is not effective. There is a grain of physiological and psychological truth in this statement. However, enjoyability of exercise is not always automatic. It must be developed.

Although enjoyment will be seen to be an important source of motivation, it is more important to learn to enjoy exercise for the sake of its effects until, like eating and sleeping, it becomes difficult to ascribe satisfaction to either the benefits or to the process alone. The appreciation of the ends will eventually transfer to an enjoyment of the means to some degree. A young man enjoys waxing his new sports car, not because of the intrinsic enjoyment of the waxing process, but because of the actual and imagined objectives that can result from owning and driving a shiny new sports car.

With this in mind, the development of physical fitness programs within modern society becomes a more realistic and attainable goal. With the realization that modern civilization has left little room for natural physical activity, intelligent beings will accept the task of exercise as well as the benefits.

Physical Fitness Components

- Aerobic Capacity
- Muscular Strength
- Muscular Endurance
- Proper Weight (percentage of fat)
- Flexibility
- Coordination
- Speed
- Muscle Balance
- Diet
- Lifestyle

2

FITNESS FACTORS

Although there is no consensus on a specific definition of physical fitness, most authorities would agree with the following sentence. Physical fitness describes the ability to cope with the daily duties of life while still having a reserve capacity for participation in enjoyable recreational activities and for meeting emergency situations. This general definition can be considered in view of the following components. While these components are interrelated, each has a distinctive feature and each contributes an essential element to physical fitness. These components will be briefly described in this chapter.

Since there is a direct relationship between your heart rate and oxygen utilization, your heart rate can be a guide to the necessary intensity of exercise. In his book *Work and the Heart*, Dr. Karvonen devised a formula for determining the rate necessary for the training effect to occur. This formula and its directions are presented in the Appendix.

AEROBIC CAPACITY

Aerobic capacity, also referred to as cardiovascular fitness, characterizes the body's ability to deliver oxygen and eliminate various by-products in the process. It involves the heart, lungs, and blood vessels and their response to contractions of the large muscle groups for relatively long periods of time.

An improvement in aerobic or cardiovascular capacity means that the body is better able to provide greater quantities of oxygen to the muscles. The muscles themselves show certain changes which make them better able to utilize the oxygen. Therefore additional energy can be released aerobically (i.e. with oxygen) and a greater capacity for prolonged exercise or physical activity results.

At any point in life a person can increase aerobic capacity through a proper conditioning program. Significant improvements are usually observed within two months. As the capacity of the heart increases, the resting heart rate slows, blood pressure reaches or maintains normal or low normal, and the efficiency of the circulation improves.

Aerobic exercise is the type which steadily supplies enough oxygen to the exercising muscles for as long as the exercise is continued without gasping for air afterward is probably aerobic. This can include bicycling, rowing, walking, running, cross-country skiing, springing, bench stepping, and rope skipping.

There is an intensity of exercise which is enough to improve aerobic capacity but is not overly strenuous. This intensity exceeds those demands usually made on sedentary persons but fall short of producing excessive fatigue, breathlessness, or mental confusion. This intensity is described as a "target zone" that is between sixty and eighty percent of one's own maximal aerobic capacity. Below sixty percent there is little fitness benefit (unless an individual has been bedridden for a prolonged period). Above eighty percent there is little added benefit with some significant disadvantages.

Frequency and Duration for Aerobic Exercise

A daily exercise routine is desirable but aerobic fitness may be enhanced by properly regulated sessions three to four days a week. Gains will be lost if more than two days elapse between sessions. Fitness rapidly deteriorates with resumption of sedentary habits. Like food and sleep, exercise cannot be stored for long.

Exercise sessions of fifteen to forty-five minutes duration usually will produce appreciable physiological and psychological effects. Activity at a lower intensity will require greater duration to produce conditioning than activity done at a higher intensity. In the initial stages of an exercise program, intensities should remain in the low range of the target zone and durations should be around twenty minutes.

MUSCULAR STRENGTH

Muscular strength refers to the contraction power of the muscles, or how much force a particular muscle group can apply in a single maximum effort. In all physical activities, muscular strength is a primary contributor and is, therefore, fundamental to success. Many ailments are also caused by insufficient muscular strength. Backache, for example, often results from weak back and abdominal muscles, and hernia can frequently be traced to weak abdominal muscles.

Strength is a specific item and must be related to body weight. A common method of scoring individual muscle strength is to divide a maximum measured exertion by one's body weight.

MUSCULAR ENDURANCE

Muscular endurance implies the capacity of a muscle or muscle group to perform repetitive actions, i.e. to perform many repetitions. Chopping, climbing, and lifting are examples of repetitive actions that require muscle endurance.

Recent research also indicates that specific changes in the chemical composition of muscle result from muscle endurance training. Such training may increase the capacities of the metabolic mechanisms for energy release in the exercised muscle cell. Muscular endurance thus may be a factor relating to increased cardiovascular endurance.

PROPER WEIGHT

Recent insurance company studies show that individuals twenty percent overweight have a death rate one-third higher than those nearer a proper weight. Heart disease, diabetes, and other ailments are significantly more common among fat individuals. Women who begin pregnancy with high initial weight are more susceptible to complications than are those of normal weight.

The determination of proper body weight can usually be assessed by a look in the mirror. However, a more accurate recommendation can be made by determining one's percentage of body fat. Ideal body fat for a man is fifteen percent and for a woman it is twenty-two percent.

The average marathon runner has a body fat percentage of about six percent, in spite of the fact that many marathon runners eat up to 5000 calories a day. This shows the effect of regular exercise on both caloric expenditure and metabolism. By increasing lean body mass, decreasing actual fat, and modifying the body's ability to metabolize fat, physical exercise becomes the most logical methodology for the acquiring of proper weight.

According to McArdle and Katch, there is evidence to suggest that controlling body fat by cutting caloric intake alone is not appropriate, nor may it be healthy. Contrary to popular mythology, fat people don't eat much more than ordinary people who have control of their body weight. So for fat people to lose weight by dieting is, in some cases, an attempt to reduce something that is already pretty low to start with—proper food intake.

FLEXIBILITY

The ability of a limb to move easily through its range of motion produces a comfortable and more efficient movement that is less likely to result in injury. Inactivity can limit the range of motion in a muscle group. In later years a sedentary individual's range of motion may be severely limited. If calcium deposits form in the joints, because they have not been moved through their full range of movement regularly, an arthritic condition may result.

Strength and endurance exercises not done in conjunction with stretching exercises can also limit flexibility by shortening the muscles. Many muscle tears, pulls, and strains occur because of a lack of flexibility.

Flexibility is achieved by moving limbs through their full range of motion and by slow and gradual stretching near the limits of movement, without pain, until the range of motion gradually increases.

COORDINATION

Coordination is the activity in which the nerves and the brain work together with the muscles as a team. The alternative to this component of fitness is clumsiness. Exercise improves coordination by developing neuro-muscular changes that improve reaction time, increase the efficiency of mechanical responses, and bring about a more rapid response to postural changes.

Inadequate coordination is responsible for many deaths and injuries, especially within the industrial environment. Improved coordination can also facilitate participation in sports activities.

MUSCLE BALANCE

Muscle balance refers to a proper ratio of strength, endurance, and flexibility among various muscle groups, especially opposing muscle groups. Specific training of one muscle group such as occurs in running does not properly train other muscle groups. When an imbalance in muscles results, the possibility for injury increases. Since imbalance injuries often result from running, and because running as a form of exercise is becoming so popular, a S.I.L.K. (Strong and Inherently Lithe Kinethesia) chart is included in the appendix. This chart, in combination with the aerobic chart, will indicate a score that will correlate with the number of miles that can be safely run with a fair assurance that overall muscle balance has been achieved.

SPEED

Speed has to do with the rapidity with which successive movement of the same kind can be performed. The only way to improve the chemical reactions that will increase speed in an activity is by performing the activity at maximum ability for increasingly longer periods of time and by specific strength training techniques. Except for sports performance, this component is only important to total fitness in certain emergency situations.

DIET

To be comprehensive, accurate, and brief in presenting an overview of nutritional principles important in maintaining optimal health and fitness is a challenging proposal. However, the essence of proper nutrition, at least that portion of the science in which there is large scale agreement among the leading authorities, can be reduced to four dietary principles:

1. Keep the intake of concentrated sugar to a minimum—especially white sugar and those products containing it.

2. Keep the intake of food additives such as preservatives, emulsifiers, coagulants, tenderizers, flavor enhancers, thickeners, bleaches, sweeteners, hydrogenated oils, artificial colorings, antioxidents, and salt, to a minimum.

3. Eat a wide variety of foods, of which sixty to seventy percent of the daily caloric intake is from raw, uncooked foods. Although many proteins, grains, and most legumes are more nutritious after cooking, a diet high in raw vegetables, fruits, seeds, and nuts will provide the highest degree of vitamins, minerals, enzymes, trace elements, and fiber.

4. In percentage of daily caloric intake, the ratio of complex carbohydrates to fats to proteins should be approximately 75: 15: 10. This is also the approximate ratio of the world's populations having the lowest incidence of heart disease, cancer, diabetes, and other debilitating diseases.

In order to determine the average proportional intake of carbohydrates, fats, and proteins the following steps should be taken. Using a gram scale, a calculator, the book *Composition of Foods*, and the form provided in the Appendix, total the figures for an entire typical day's food consumption. By doing this once or twice a month sufficient knowledge and awareness can be gained to modify a diet appropriately.

In addition to the four major dietary guidelines listed above, two others are suggested by the nutritionist Paalo Airola that are worthy of note. Dr. Airola contends that "systematic undereating" is one of the most important dietary considerations applicable to the healthy populations of the world. He also recommends very moderate vitamin and mineral supplements (naturally derived only) to make up for the loss of nutrients in foods resulting from soil condition, pollution, and storage.

LIFESTYLE

Although lifestyle encompasses all of the components of physical fitness, it is important to recognize those basic considerations that have not yet been mentioned. These include:

- smoking
- drug abuse, including alcohol, prescription, and nonprescription drugs.
- proper rest
- stress reduction; the ability to cope successfully with life's stresses
- attitude and philosophy of life; the establishment of proper priorities, self-esteem, and the striving toward one's full positive potentiality.

In organizing any fitness program for adults, special attention should be given to the participants back. It is probable that the majority of all prospective participants in a beginning fitness program will have lower back pain. If not properly treated before a regular exercise program, back pain can worsen with exercise and a participant is likely to withdraw from the program.

PART TWO:
FITNESS PROGRAMS
FOR BUSINESS
AND INDUSTRY

3

DOLLARS FOR YOUR DEEDS

A truism too important to mention is often completely ignored. Less than 2.5 percent of our total national expenditure for health care is for prevention, and a similarly insignificant amount is targeted for fitness education and opportunities. The result is an annual medical bill of over 200 billion dollars!

Forty percent of this astronomical bill is paid by the business community. It is this segment of society where the most logical acceptance of the responsibility for health maintenance programs should exist. Dr. Mark Bond, Corporate Medical Director for AT & T, and Industrial Consultant for the California Health Research Foundation, is in agreement:

> As major contributors to the considerable annual health care expenditure, the most sensible corporate position would be a shift from the current passive role, wherein companies reluctantly spend more on health care services without noticeable reward, to an active role involving cost control and health promotion programs. It is apparent that our current emphasis on medical coverage as an employee benefit has de-emphasized the customary corporate policy of cost-effectiveness, and allowed this unchecked expense to be accepted as a fact of life. It is in fact a matter of life and death.

Economic efficiency is a key factor in most business decisions. Employee fitness programs are not only efficient, if properly implemented, they are also economically productive. They can be responsible for improvements in morale and a resultant improvement in the quality of goods or services. They can reduce absenteeism and premature retirement of valuable personnel.

A fitness program is also good for a company's image. For many companies employee fitness programs and facilities are major attractions to prospective executives during the process of recruitment. The same image is also good public relations. A concern about the welfare of employees implies a concern for the well-being and satisfaction of its customer.

To be effective any attempt to reduce medical and disability costs in business and industry must stress prevention. Any serious effort to improve the living and working habits of employees and executives must involve a commitment to physical fitness.

The opportunity to reintroduce physical activity into the work environment is exciting. The time requirements are minimal and the eventual payoff should be indisputable.

The Proof Rationale

There is much evidence that suggests that the economic return from an employee fitness program far exceeds the investment. The cogency of this evidence has compelled many business leaders to develop fitness programs but the majority of decision makers are not yet convinced.

The question of proof has historically provided the testing grounds for progress. An innovation had to penetrate the status quo barrier before it would be investigated. It had to withstand the attacks of the defenders of the status quo before it would be recognized. It had to pass the test of time before it would be accepted. As a result the community at large could be confident that the innovation was a step in the right direction.

This traditional process of determining validity has also had its tragic repercussions. Legislators were once petitioned by farsighted and concerned citizens to pass laws prohibiting wood-shake roofs on attached apartments. Many people burned to death in conflagrations before such laws were passed. Vaccines were invented to prevent disease. Many people died needlessly before the medical community began using the vaccines.

Similarly, health experts are recommending physical fitness programs to decrease morbidity, mortality, and the related costs to business and society. But the recommendations are muffled by the calls for more proof and the rapid deterioration of health and productivity in the country are the result.

The hesitation to acknowledge that employee fitness programs are economically efficient is not just related to the lack of empirical conclusions from longitudinal studies. It also has to do with the long-term nature of prevention. A program designed to prevent something from happening in the future may seem too vague to a pragmatic businessman. On the other hand, an insurance policy that will afford a cure for an ill employee is a more visible reality to such a person. It doesn't matter that a pound of cure is more expensive and less valuable than an ounce of prevention. What seems to matter is that the former is more obvious and less likely to be lost amidst the daily rituals of business.

In terms of finding out if physical fitness really does have a money payoff, there has been a failure of common sense. High degrees of probability have been ignored for want of statistically significant, empirical data. Specific proof demands less risk than logical deduction. If a manager has infallible data that corporate fitness programs decreased absenteeism, disabilities, premature retirements, insurance premiums, and increased productivity by significant amounts, even the most careful decision maker would implement employee fitness programs. But if such a conclusion has to be based on reasoning, a commitment to a fitness program might require courage and far-sightedness. An example of such reasoning might be as follows.

People who exercise properly are not apt to be overfat. People who are not overfat have fewer back injuries. People who have fewer back injuries are less likely to be disabled. People who are less likely to be disabled are less likely to incur compensation costs to an employer. Therefore, a fitness program that encourages people to exercise properly is a sound investment.

There is sufficient logic in this reasoning but not sufficient traditional "proof." There are, however, business leaders who do follow the tide of such logic. Sagaciousness and courage to take risks are part of the qualities of a progressive businessman. This is why many responsible companies have made significant commitments to employee fitness. While many of these programs have not yet been found cost-effective in terms of their initial investment, their long-term benefits may be significant. These companies are at least not going to risk the cost of waiting for further proof. And while large investments are not necessary for effective fitness programs, many of these companies have been willing to invest millions of dollars in the gamble.

While the doctrine of common sense should be applied in considering employee fitness programs, there is still a need for more statistical evidence. There is an important need for better organized protocols, better use of statistics, and a pooling of research materials and information. In the meantime, this section of the book will provide the reader with the most significant evidence for establishing a credible rationale for the development of fitness programs in business and industry.

The Pioneers

One reasonable rationale for implementing employee fitness programs may simply be the observation that many other reputable and responsible companies have already taken the step. More than three hundred major companies employ full-time fitness directors, and hundreds of others have more modest programs. The list of private firms committed to employee fitness exemplifies the ability to make responsible managerial decisions regarding products as well as people. Arco, Chase Manhattan, Western Electric, Exxon, General Foods, Firestone, Pepsico, Goodyear, Phillips Petroleum, Boeing, Xerox, Rockwell International, Merrill Lynch, Kimberly-Clark, Mobil, Weyerhaeuser, and Johns-Mansville are just a few.

In addition, several insurance companies have implemented employee fitness programs. The conservative nature of insurance companies in combination with their reliance on mortality and morbidity statistics and research make this an important consideration. The Board of Directors at Metropolitan Life, John Hancock Mutual Life, Sentry Insurance, Occidental Life, and Life of Georgia concluded that employee fitness programs were economically productive. Howard Dobbs, chairman of the board of Life of Georgia, estimates that the increased life expectancy of key staff is enough to cover the investment cost involved.

Major governmental agencies have also considered the cost-effective nature of employee fitness programs. The highly successful NASA employee fitness program demonstrated the rationale for public funding of employee fitness programs and other agencies are following suit. The Senate is including a multi-purpose athletic room in its extension to the Dirksen Building. The Environmental Protection Agency, the Smithsonian Institution, and the Departments of Transportation and Justice provide their employees with time and facilities for exercise. Although these programs are just a beginning, the President's Council on Physical Fitness is trying to encourage the development of employee fitness programs for all American workers (employees), whether in the public or private sector.

Another group that is developing the employee fitness frontier is the American Association of Fitness Directors in Business and Industry (AAFDBI). Organized at a volleyball game by a small group of fitness leaders and exercise physiologists, membership in the AAFDBI has grown from the original thirty-nine members in 1975 to more than one thousand in 1979. An affiliate of the President's Council on Physical Fitness and Sports, the AAFDBI is an excellent clearinghouse for collecting and distributing information regarding employee fitness programs.

It is somewhat remarkable that employee fitness has remained a frontier until so recent a moment in history. The first comprehensive description of a major corporate physical fitness program wasn't published until 1974. The publication in the *Journal of Occupational Medicine* described the Exxon fitness program in New York. Most of the major attempts to improve productivity and reduce medical costs with fitness programs have occurred within the past decade.

With a few exceptions, most employee fitness programs prior to 1970 emphasized the recreational aspect of fitness as opposed to the physical aspect. One notable exception was the National Cash Register Company. In 1894, John H. Patterson of the National Cash Register Company in Dayton, Ohio, introduced morning and afternoon exercise breaks for his employees. This may be the first employee exercise program in American history. In 1904 Mr. Patterson installed a gym on the fourth floor and in 1911 he opened a 325-acre park for his employees.

There were other companies with programs that resulted in improved physical fitness, but the improvements were often restricted to talented sports participants and were often short-lived or seasonal. For example, the Indian Packing Company in Green Bay, Wisconsin sponsored an employee football team that became known as the Green Bay Packers. Until recently industrial fitness programs were comprised of bowling leagues, softball leagues, and the like. In 1941 the National Industrial Recreation Association (NIRA), was founded to stimulate interest in recreation for employees, i.e. sports, travel, and hobbies, but it finds itself now in the role of a physical fitness advisor to many companies.

The pioneering efforts in employee fitness must be respected in lieu of the cultural influences on traditional American work ethics. Rapid technological advancements, the employer-employee dichotomy, traditional health care practices, and other factors have created a difficult environment. (These influences will be discussed in detail in Chapter 4). Nonetheless, employee fitness programs emphasizing health and recreation and its relation to economic efficiency have been a reality in foreign countries for many years. Japanese exercise breaks, Russian industrial fitness programs, and European health clubs are an integral part of the working cycle.

Absenteeism

If neither the recognition of precedents nor the application of general fitness data to economic efficiency is sufficiently motivating, then every effort must be made to provide as much specific evidence as possible. One of the most common claims that employee fitness programs are effective is that they can reduce absenteeism. Although many longitudinal studies are just beginning, there is some significant evidence already available that this might indeed be a valid incentive

In the *British Journal of Industrial Medicine*, Dr. V. Linden noted that the absence pattern of customs officers was directly related to their maximal oxygen uptake. According to the President's Council on Physical Fitness and Sports, "physically fit employees are directly related to higher production, positive problem solving, cooperation, creative thinking, and reduced absenteeism." Even without specific evidence, if the first four claims were valid it would follow that an employee would be absent less frequently.

A survey at the Occidental Life Insurance Company of California in 1978 showed that regular users of the company gym are absent only half as often as nonusers, according to Bob Rush, group sales manager and supervisor of the fitness program there. When a Goodyear plant in Norrkopking, Sweden introduced an employee fitness program, absenteeism among participants also fell by nearly half.

These two results may be exceptional but even a modest reduction would yield very substantial savings. Absenteeism in the executive branch of government alone costs 1.34 billion dollars and accounts for twenty-five million lost workdays every year.

A study of absenteeism by the Public Health Service cited "habitual inactivity" as a prime factor in the high absenteeism. In its words, "Habitual inactivity is thought to contribute to hypertension, chronic fatigue and resulting physical inefficiency, premature aging, the poor musculature and lack of flexibility which are the major causes of lower back pain and injury, mental tension, coronary heart disease, obesity, and other major causes of absenteeism. By contrast studies have reported that regular exercise can reduce or reverse these manifestations."

Perhaps the most significant tangible evidence relating fitness to absenteeism comes from the U.S.S.R. In his thesis on the effect of physical exercises on health and economic efficiency, Professor V. Pravosudov of the Iesgaft State Institute of Physical Culture in Leningrad discussed data concerning the sick rate of individuals involved in regular physical fitness programs. One conclusion, based on a study by K. Smirnov, was that persons taking part in fitness activity consulted doctors four times less than those not engaged in physical training, and their sick rate with temporary lost ability to work made up twenty-two percent of these consultations compared to sixty percent of the second group.

In his thesis, Professor Pravosudov presents several longitudinal studies that compared the frequency of primary cases of consulting a doctor on the occasion of the flu, acute catarrhal (inflammation of mucous membranes), and other diseases between exercisers and non-exercisers. The facts indicated that the exercisers were less subject to complications, there was a lower probability of the transition of illnesses to chronic diseases, they were sick less often, and their ill-nesses passed more rapidly.

Sociological research among the workers of Russia reaffirmed these findings. Workers regularly practicing physical exercises, according to a compilation of six separate studies, fell ill three to four times less than those of the same age not engaged in regular physical activity. As for the middle-aged and elderly people, this difference increased to six to eight times. The workers taking part in fitness programs missed fewer days work. These studies included industrial, office, and professional workers. Furthermore, the studies indicated that the physical activity participation of workers decreases the losses on "sick-bulletin" days on the average of three to five days a year for one worker. In Russia this means an extra use of 140 million men days in industry and millions of roubles of extra output.

Although the conclusions regarding absenteeism in this country are based on smaller numbers and more short-term studies, there are still some significant findings. For example, Criss Cadillac of Provi-dence reported that the fifteen of sixty-five employees that enrolled in their fitness program have been absent on the average of three days per year less than those not enrolled. New York Telephone estimated an annual savings from reduced absenteeism of 30,000 dol-lars at just one work site. Another program in Albany, New York in-volved a five year program involving 847 employees. The program was conducted and evaluated by Dr. Larry A. Bjurstrom and was financed by federal, state, and employee contributions. The results were a significant reduction in heart disease risk factors (cholesterol, obesity, smoking habits, triglycerides), amelioration of many health problems and a significant reduction in employee absenteeism.

Productivity

Absenteeism is one factor in determining the economic efficiency of employee fitness programs, but what happens at a workplace even when employees are present may be even more significant. The ques-tion of human productivity is of utmost importance both socially and economically. Business and industry pay when employees lack enthusiasm and vitality, and so do the employees. A physically fit and productive employee stays on the job longer, rises faster in a firm, thinks more clearly and operates more safely, gets along better with co-workers, and generally gets more out of the job.

In the introduction to his book, J.D. Hackett had the following paragraph:

"Chickens, racehorses, and circus monkeys are fed, housed, trained, and kept up to the highest physical pitch in order to secure a full return from them as producers in their respective functions. The same principle applies to human beings; increased production cannot be expected from workers unless some attention is paid to their physical needs."

Every employer claims that his people are his greatest asset, but workers remain the least tapped resources within most companies. Productivity of an employee involves a good deal more than the ability to show up.

One of the pioneering experiments in this country to show that fitness programs can improve productivity began in 1968 at the Washington headquarters of the National Aeronautics and Space Administration. In cooperation with the Heart Disease and Stroke Control Program of the Public Health Service, the space agency provided a thrice-weekly exercise program for 259 executives, men aged thirty-five to fifty-five. After a year, the participants completed questionnaires and underwent a thorough medical examination.

The findings were impressive. Half the regular participants reported improved on the job performance and better attitudes toward their work. Twelve percent of the sporadic participants reported similar performance and attitude improvement. Nearly all the regular participants said they felt better; eighty-nine percent reported improved stamina, and nearly half that number reported sounder sleep. More than sixty percent lost weight. Many participants quit smoking or cut down, and nearly half said they were paying more attention to their diets. Most important, there was a "highly consistent and positive relationship" between the perceived benefits of the program and the results of medical tests. Those who reported improved stamina showed marked improvements in cardiovascular performance, as measured by treadmill tests.

Evidence demonstrating a relationship between higher productivity and levels of fitness is also prevalent in the Soviet Union. Investigations carried out at various enterprises in Russian towns distinctly showed that, other things being equal, the "worker-athletes" had a higher working capacity, the rate of their output standard being two to five percent and sometimes ten to fifteen percent higher than with non-exercisers.

More pronounced distinctions were manifested where manual labor prevailed, and improvements were noted among office workers as well. The Russian researchers pointed out that physical exercises produce a "favorable influence on mental labor productivity." The researches carried out in schools and higher education establishments in the U.S.S.R. showed that regular physical activity resulted in students making better progress. They also found out that a steady mental working capacity during the whole day and the likeness in the course of the processes of rehabilitation after big manual and mental loads.

While making a careful study of the physical training program at a Siberian branch of the Academy of Sciences of the Soviet Union, E. Podalko (1977) showed in his thesis that high physical training activity of the scientists and the state of their health, as well as the working capacity of their creative activity, are in close connection. Further Soviet studies show that setting up exercises at work among industrial, office, and professional workers helps to keep the working capacity at a high level up to the end of the working day. In the Council of Europe's "Sport for All" publication, reference is made to a number of studies in a chapter, "Physical Activity and Capacity for Work." For example, errors of women textile workers decreased thirty-one percent in a group receiving regular exercise breaks.

It has also been verified that the mere participatory effect of an employee fitness program can stimulate and enhance productivity. Employee fitness programs are an excellent opportunity for inter-relationships between management and submanagement. In some companies they represent the only available cooperative enterprise for all workers. When the programs are set up in accordance with the guidelines in this book, a fitness program promotes that concept that everyone is contributing to the life of a business in a sense that goes beyond the assigned duties and tasks of a particular job.

Many studies have shown that increased participation among employees in the affairs of a business can increase productivity. In a controlled comparison of managerial and cooperative enterprises in Israel, Melman found that the cooperative enterprises had higher median sales per man hour than did managerial enterprises of similar size and comparable products. They also had higher productivity of capital, larger net profit per production worker, and lower administrative costs.

In an evaluation of Swedish industry, Karlsson came to a similar conclusion. "Productivity and economic performance of those firms involved in making changes that increased worker participation improved. This improvement seems attributable to the increased flexibility and feeling of importance that the employees associate with such participation. Substantial improvements in reported job satisfaction were recorded that confirmed this."

The Japanese experience further supports this hypothesis. The high productivity of Japanese industry is obvious to the entire world. The production philosophy of Toyota is representative. They place a great deal of importance on good human relations. They actively promote participation in group activities under the slogan, "Discover a different you in sports and hobbies." Toyota management believes that such activities help the workers start each new day with renewed enthusiasm as well as to strengthen their sense of participation in the company.

An example of Toyota commitment to this philosophy is their athletic facilities. The Toyota Sports Center was constructed at a total cost of fourteen million dollars. Open to the general public as well as to employees and their families, the center serves the recreational and health needs of the local community and promotes good human relations among, and the physical health of, Toyota employees.

The result is one of the most productive companies in the world. Using the formula of number of vehicles produced divided by the number of employees, the productivity factor of Toyota is 51.3 compared to 9.6 for General Motors and 12.0 for Ford. In a meeting of the President's Council on Physical Fitness and Sports, President Carter remarked on the low productivity of American workers in comparison to the 1940s when America was second in world productivity only to West Germany. He then queried whether or not it was coincidental that the Japanese, who have committed themselves to employee fitness, were leaders in both longevity of life and in productivity of goods.

Although it seems on the basis of the above information that improved fitness means improved productivity, research on the subject is still not conclusive. The balance of data, however, suggests improved productivity. As will be seen in the next chapter, the prevention of one heart attack may be worth twice any expected increase in actual production. Besides, a more longitudinal study may have shown an improvement. A good example of this possibility is illustrated by the following anecdote.

Rick Winners, a top salaried salesman for a national company, was suffering from ulcers, nervous disorders, and the harmful effects of cigarette smoking. After participating in a personal fitness program for about one year, he cured his ulcer, quit smoking, improved his appearance, and regained his sense of vitality. Although he maintained a satisfactory sales quota, he eased off the pressure for an extremely high income in exchange for the time to take care of his health.

During his annual evaluation interview Rick's boss asked him the usual question, "What did you do for the company this year?"

Rick answered proudly, "I lost ten pounds of fat, quit smoking, and started running every day."

The following year, he doubled his sales.

Medical Costs

The most obvious relationship between physical fitness and economic efficiency has to do with the reduction of health care costs. Actuarial data available to the many insurance companies that have implemented employee fitness programs reveal the value of maintaining a low-risk lifestyle. George Schilser, fitness director of the Life Insurance Company of Georgia stated, "We deal in health and mortality statistics every day. We know that obese people get more diabetes, hypertension, and heart disease than slim ones, and that out of shape individuals get sick more often than their fit colleagues. Our management feels that keeping employees healthy is plain good business."

Poor fitness contributes directly to the rising cost of health insurance. General Motors, for example, now spends 825 million dollars for its employee health plan. That is more than it spends to purchase steel from U.S. Steel, its principal supplier. In 1976, health benefits added 175 dollars to the price of every car and truck manufactured by them. For all industries, the backache alone, usually a result of neglected muscles, accounts for a quarter billion dollars in workmen's compensation claims annually.

Other health care costs relating to inadequate levels of fitness are equally staggering. North American Rockwell estimates an annual cost per alcoholic employee of more than fifty thousand dollars. United California Bank of Los Angeles estimates an annual cost for alcoholism in a work force of ten thousand employees at one million dollars! According to U.S. Health statistics, disability insurance in 1950 was two million, and it has risen to 103 million in 1977. Workers compensation went from 193 million in 1950 to 2,609,000,000 in 1977!

An insurers premium charges for an employee group depend partly on the amount the insurer had to pay out for the group's medical expenses in the past. Kimberly Clark, who recently put together a 2.5 million dollar exercise program, had premiums costing

14.3 million dollars in 1977, seventy-five percent higher than they were in 1973 to cover 150,000 employees. At Ford Motor Company health insurance is their most expensive fringe benefit. It went from 450 million in 1977 to 600 million in 1978.

A recently completed report in the Province of Ontario relates the physical fitness of participants to their health care costs, as measured by the frequency of doctor and hospital visits, number of days off work due to ill health, and the amount of physician claims made under the Ontario Health Insurance Plan. Among the conclusions of this important study are the following:

1. People with higher levels of physical fitness tend to have lower medical claims.

2. An estimated reduction of thirty-one million dollars in medical claims could be expected if all adults aged twenty to sixty-nine years were of at least average physical fitness.

In the near future, insurance rates will be discounted to fit individuals and companies with fit employees. One company, Occidental Life of North Carolina, has already started advertising a twenty percent discount on all life insurance rates for fit individuals. The ad pictures a fit looking executive carrying an obese, cigarette smoking executive on his shoulders with the caption, "You may be in prime condition, but you're still shouldering overweight insurance rates." The program is limited to active people who regularly participate in aerobic related exercise programs at least three times a week for twenty minute durations.

In order for a company to appreciate the cost and extent of its medical claims, the managers should study the use of medical facilities, the amount of medical claims, disabilities, and premature retirement. The American Heart Association estimates that the cost of replacing employees who have had a heart attack is 700 million dollars annually.

Perhaps the most significant public statement regarding the need and effectiveness of fitness programs in curbing the cost of health care comes from the 1978 H.E.W. convention, where it was announced that programs promoting health maintenance and disease prevention would be exempt from the President's wage and price control. Whether or not this will provide an actual incentive for such programs remains to be seen. It does indicate the economic importance attached to this approach to reducing medical costs.

Program Costs

"The beauty of employee fitness programs is that they can be remarkably inexpensive," says Dr. Richard O. Keelor, director of Program Development for the President's Council on Physical Fitness and Sports. "Not all companies can afford a spacious gymnasium but elaborate equipment is not essential."

This indeed is another great virtue of employee fitness programs. An effective fitness program is not dependent upon expensive facilities. Kimberly Clark's 2.5 million dollar fitness center and Xerox's two million dollar facility provide a luxurious environment and many convenient exercise alternatives and amenities. These things can play an important role in motivating people to exercise and offer an impressive example of an employee fitness commitment. However, the success of these programs is no greater than that demonstrated by the fitness programs of Memorex or ESL Inc., where there is no facility at all.

As will become clear throughout these pages, the key to a successful program is not facilities. It is leadership and organization. A program can be just as successful giving company time to exercise beside a desk as spending thousands equipping gyms and paying full-time fitness directors.

George Schisler, director of physical fitness and recreation at the Life Insurance Company of Georgia, agrees. He feels that the people and the methodologies involved in implementing a fitness program in industry are more important that the investment in the training and exercise facilities. "All I need is a room with some mats to double or triple the strength measurements, flexibility, and well-being of a participant," he says. "Firms immediately consider what kind of equipment they need rather than the leaders who will direct the program."

The first cost consideration should therefore be directed at who will develop and implement the program. There may be an individual in the business who qualifies as a fitness director. (A special section will describe leadership qualifications.) A person with leadership capabilities could also be trained as a fitness specialist for a reasonable time and money commitment. Part-time fitness instructors can be hired at reasonable rates. One company, Scully-Emhart, entered into a contractual relationship between a Y.M.C.A. and eighty employees for an employee fitness program at a total cost of ten thousand dollars. Another initiated a pilot program by simply hiring a fitness specialist to lecture and administer basic fitness tests at a cost of eighty-five dollars per employee. Weyerhaeusers' program is run on a club basis with a nine dollar a month subscription fee.

A wide variety of fitness programs and facilities will be discussed in detail later, but it is important for the reader to appreciate the fact that an exorbitant out-of-pocket investment is not a prerequisite for a fitness program. Any long-term expenditure can be cost-effective based on an evaluation of the pilot program. And any successful program, regardless of the cost, will result in a significant return.

Next to facilities and management, liabilities connected with the fitness program present another possible cost. Any injury sustained in a fitness program is covered by workman's compensation and a number of exercise related claims could negate short-term cost effectiveness of a fitness program. A risk analysis would be correct in studying this aspect.

The prospect of such liabilities being significant, however, is slight if the program guidelines recommended in this book are followed. Any minor injuries that may be sustained in the beginning stages of a program are not comparable economically to the prevention of longer term disabilities. Any company risk analyst who is aware of these guidelines and the potential return from the fitness program should have little trouble recommending approval of a proposed program.

The Greatest Asset

The most important lesson of this section is the realization that people are an organization's greatest asset. This recurring theme is the essential realization necessary to spark fitness programs in business and industry. Managers must remember that work is done by a human being.

Working therefore involves physiology, psychology, social life, and personality as well as economics.

It is also important that this realization be manifested in the image of a fitness program. Employees should believe that the fitness program represents a concern for their own well-being and not just the economic productivity of the company. The image a company should try to project isn't the reduction of absenteeism, improvement of morale, or cost reductions in health insurance. It is the one-to-one concern over helping the employee live and work at his best.

Jim Daineill, Vice President of North American Rockwell, bespeaks this sentiment. "The greatest asset our company has," he says, "is its people, every last one of them. We don't want to lose them through illness and heart attacks, and we're not going to if we can help it."

W.W. Keeler, Chairman of the Board of Phillips Petroleum Company, concurs. "For most of us, the benefits of a physical conditioning program go beyond more productive individuals. They live longer and happier. When we consider the investment our companies have in people, and our reliance on their skills and experience, it is clear that the longevity of employees is a real benefit to our organization."

R.H. Dobbs, Sr., President of the Life Insurance Company of Georgia, also believes, "It's good business to keep our key personnel healthy. It means less time loss. I'm also convinced that if we can add a few years to our employees' lives it will mean a tremendous financial saving as well as the satisfaction of knowing that our people feel better, stay in better humor, and can handle people better because of their participation in our fitness program."

An employee fitness program indeed has a great influence on both social and economic well-being. The widely acclaimed National Aeronautics and Space Administration fitness project reported many benefits resulting from its program. Program participants reported the following effects in descending order of frequency:

- decrease in food consumption
- more positive work attitude
- less stress and tension
- improved work performance
- more selective in kind of food consumed
- increased physical activity beyond the program
- expanded recreational activities
- more adequate sleep and rest
- reduction in smoking
- improved sexual relations

In general, the participant's wife and his work associates were also mentioned as an extension of the benefits. An individual's participation in the program served as a model and incentive for health behavior change among those persons with whom he or she related most directly. This indirect effect also enhanced the total well-being of an employee if those he lives and works with are also happier and healthier.

The concern of an employer for the well-being of his employees away from work as well as at work has another implication. By educating people in the workplace about safety and health and by making them more fit, more alert and more responsive, many off-duty disabilities can be prevented. The National Safety Council says that seventy percent of accidental deaths occur away from work, as well as fifty percent of accidental disabilities. In 1978 one person in every four had an accident that accounted for a total of ninety-eight million lost workdays!

Similarly, employee physical fitness programs can reduce health problems related to drug abuse. A significant finding from fitness program research at Xerox was the tendency of participants to cut down on alcohol and tobacco or to quit the habits altogether. People had an increased ability to handle crisis situations without the aid of drugs.

A similar conclusion was verified by Dr. Joyce Brothers and Dr. Herbert DeVries in independent studies comparing the electrical activity in the muscles before and after exercise and before and after a tranquilizer. It was found that seventeen minutes of exercise had the same effect as a frequently prescribed dosage of valium.

Considering the fact that alcohol abusers are responsible for five times as many compensation costs as non-abusers, that alcoholism costs industry twenty billion dollars in lost work time, and that Americans spend more than 100 million dollars annually on valium alone, a reduction in drug abuse via a fitness program represents another valuable protection aspect of a company's most important assets.

Thus an employee fitness program affects in some degree all of the life's activities of the company's most valuable asset. It follows that all of the employee's activities are in some way brought into the working environment. Physical fitness for this employee means the ability to carry out daily tasks with vigor and alertness without undue fatigue and with ample energy to enjoy leisure time pursuits and meet unforeseen emergencies. As a result an employee will be less likely to suffer an industrial accident or an accident away from work, and will be happier and more productive.

An investment in the human asset results in a payoff difficult to match with any other single innovation. There is an immediate reduction in overhead costs due to chronic unfitness of employees. A company will acquire a reputation for caring about the human side of the workplace. This image will attract and keep good people. And there will be an interaction between employers and employees that will be conducive to improved morale and efficiency.

Dr. Richard Morrison, who pioneered the physical fitness program for the space division of the North American Rockwell Corporation, sums it up as follows: "If our program saves the health of just a few employees, and I believe the score is already much higher than that, the cost will have been more than repaid. A healthier employee is a more effective employee. He contributes more when he is on the job, and because he's healthier he spends less time off the job. And to the extent the program reduces the occasions for replacing executives, it pays its way and nets incalculable dividends in moral and human hope."

Why fitness? It adds quality and dimension to life and that means happier people. It improves health and that means consistently higher performance levels and reduced medical costs. And that means good business!

4

BROACHING THE BARRIERS

Despite the evidence that fitness is a major factor in social and economic well-being, the fitness movement has great opposition. The opposition exists deep within the foundation of society; lurking within social mores, individual psyches, business traditions, and national institutions. Before business leaders can implement the fitness priority successfully, they must first recognize and evaluate basic cultural contradictions.

The contradictions are subtle, but powerful. The advertising media have managed to associate cigarettes, alcohol, and Coca-Cola with healthy outdoor activities. An interest in national sports has replaced athletic participation. A medical profession trained in disease care claims national leadership in the area of health care. Educators cry for change but teach only how to maintain the status quo.

Furthermore there are intentional enemies to the acquisition of health. For the sake of profit food is poisoned, air is polluted, and children are misled. For the sake of power, legislators disguise the truth. For the lack of information, courage, and wisdom, "nations have passed away."

In each section of this book there will be a description of those barriers that most influence the population that is targeted. It should be noted, however, that a barrier to fitness in one population may be a barrier to fitness for another. The inter-relationship between business and industry, children, older people, and communities is obvious. All are influenced by government, education, medicine, media, the profit motive, and cultural and personal values.

It is going to be difficult to encourage the re-evaluation of such forces, but lifestyle education must include those factors. Iatrogenic examples and governmental hypocrisy are illustrated not to shock the reader but to stimulate an awareness of those factors that can cause a fitness program to fail before it begins. The foundation that is supporting poor health must be reconstructed. Such is the nature of a revolution if it is to be successful.

The more profound cultural and political barriers referred to above are not as applicable in discussing business and industry fitness programs as they are in discussing programs for children, older persons, and communities at large. Although businessmen are still subjectively influenced by such considerations, they are more objectively motivated within the business structure. In this section the barriers that will be discussed relate to management, values and emotions, legal considerations, the medical department, and systems and regulations.

Rigidity and Risk

The basic barrier to fitness program implementation in business and industry has to do with the lack of an understanding of the impact of exercise and health education on the business situation. According to Douglas R. Brown, associate professor at Cornell University's graduate school of business and public administration, many company managers are overwhelmed by the complexity of the health care cost problem. He refers to executives like John Woodlock, Vice President and Treasurer of Continental Air Lines who asserts in frustration, "There's nothing more that we can do other than ask our people to be more discreet in how they spend their health dollars."

The impact of fitness on business has been presented, but without efficient management the information may be useless. A common example of inefficient management is the tendency to reflect on attitudes rather than analysis. Managers usually think only in terms of the traditional dimensions of the business world; space, money, and time. By remaining within this dimension, a manager believes he is eliminating risk.

To try to eliminate risk in a business enterprise is futile. Risk is an inherent aspect of any commitment of present resources to future expectations. An attempt to eliminate such risks is irrational and can result in the greatest risk of all, rigidity.

According to Malek, such rigidity is common among many top managers in the United States. He states that management skills have seldom been given prime consideration in selecting people for high level posts. Most have had little training or experience in management. Many are narrow, functional specialists rather than managerial generalists. As a result, top management often becomes committed to a singular program or discipline and may be unwilling to consider innovations such as an employee fitness program.

If fitness programs are to become a solution to the applicable problems of business and industry, managers will have to broaden their scope of expertise and awareness. They will have to acquire an overview that will reveal the many components within business that need recognition.

Adversary Barrier

One of the most dramatic components that is in need of recognition from management is the "happy people" component. This concept maintains that a workplace that takes some responsibility for an employee's social welfare will reap the benefits of a higher level of work performance, better attendance, and less turnover.

Traditional approaches to the managing of people have not focused on people as a resource, but as problems, procedures, and costs. In fact, people have often been the least utilized resource in many business organizations. According to Drucker, the quality of life of an employee and his community is a major task area for management. The public is already demanding that business be responsible for the effect of its products on the social and physical environment. The next call may demand some responsibility for the social and physical well-being of its employees.

This concept is important because a fitness program, if it is to be successful, will require conciliation between employee and employers. The traditional dichotomy between labor and management will stifle any attempt at an employee fitness program. Without an indication that there is a sincere concern for the health of the employee, a fitness program may be seen as another means for control of the employee and his security.

Historically, management has not often appreciated the "happy people" concept of work. Sweat shops, child labor, and poor working conditions have given sad testimony to the dehumanization of workers. To a different degree, the adversary posture between employers and employees still exists. Management's concern for production has overshadowed its concern for people. As a result workers begin to lose self-esteem and become dissatisfied with their work. This management "versus" worker syndrome cannot promote optimal productivity. In fact, according to a report by the Department of Labor, job dissatisfaction is a major cause of debilitation and is the greatest single predictor of work longevity.

Although one of the advantages of implementing a fitness program is to improve employer-employee relations, the adversary image of management must be somewhat overcome before a fitness program concept is initiated. With such prevailing attitudes, employee attitudes towards the fitness program could be negative and the success of the program is doomed.

One of the ways to implement the "happy people" priority is to allow for increased worker participation in managerial tasks. Programs can be initiated that begin to give workers more control over matters that directly affect their work, i.e., work methods, work speed, etc. The role of supervisors can be modified to one of an advisory nature. Perhaps workers could be given opportunities to participate in corporate decision making. Managers could occasionally take a seat on the assembly line. All in all, communication can be transformed into a two-way street.

Once such an environment is established and employees understand that there is a sincere effort on the part of management to recognize their value and respect their role, the foundation for the fitness program will be laid. With the realization that management is concerned with the employee's welfare, the acceptance of a fitness program is more likely. The program will then be a logical extension of the new managerial philosophy instead of being an extension of the adversary posture. It will be viewed as a benefit instead of a threat.

With such a managerial strategy in effect, management will not only have overcome a barrier to the implementation of a fitness program, it will also be taking a progressive step toward accomplishing the entrepreneurial tasks of the organization.

Fitness versus Recreation

The traditional existence of company recreation programs can also pose a barrier to "selling" or organizing a fitness program. Even businesses most guilty of the adversary posture often have sponsored recreational programs, e.g., picnics, bowling leagues, or softball, for employees as a token acknowledgment of the "happy people" philosophy. Management spends substantial sums on "recreational" type programs that are used by a minority of employees (probably those least in need of physical activity). The money is spent to appease the employee as a sign of good relations. Then, when fitness programs are brought up, many managers think of them only in terms of being additional recreational programs and not worth the managerial attention that they deserve.

Advocates of exercise have been saying for years that physical fitness programs are of a much different nature than typical recreation programs such as group sports, dances, and so forth. It is this difference that makes the fitness programs so important and it is imperative that management be informed as to the difference.

In those instances where recreational programs do not actually reflect a sincere "happy people" strategy, or where the programs are ineffective in satisfying the majority of people, the programs should be reevaluated and substituted with planning efforts that more accurately reflect a concern for the welfare of the employee. In some instances the money saved could be used for the development of the fitness program.

The Visibility Problem

Another managerial barrier to the development of fitness programs has to do with management's frequent unwillingness to support actions which cannot be measured in the short term with quantifiable indexes. Although a fitness program can reflect positive results in terms of health and physiology in the short term, the program's effect on productivity and absenteeism is a long-term gamble. In this case it is not the gamble that is the barrier but the apparent lack of quantifiable measurements.

Short-term visibility is a common criterion for program approval. A good example are alcohol programs. Alcohol abusers cost business and industry millions of dollars. An estimated ten percent of the work force are alcohol abusers. The problem is very visible, and the typical program offers visible and immediate solutions. It does not matter that the solutions are often only temporary, only that they are rapid and visible.

Another example is the commercial coronary rehabilitation programs that are currently gaining popularity in business and industry. Here again the problem is visible; a top executive has actually had a heart attack. The company needs to have him back in the saddle, and within a few short months, many heart attack victims are able to return to work healthier than before they had their heart attack.

The coronary rehabilitation programs are indeed nothing more than physical fitness programs for people who have had heart attacks. But the visibility of the problem and the remedy is much greater than is the case with a population that has not yet had the heart attack.

The answer to this problem is, again, to educate the manager who requires rapid feedback to accept the physiological improvements in blood pressure, heart rate, body fat, and oxygen uptake that can result in the short term from a fitness program. It is wiser, safer, and more economical to provide fitness programs for populations of employees at risk for heart disease than exclusively for employees who have already had heart attacks.

Emotional Barriers

Human nature, values, and emotions are often the most difficult barriers to the acceptance and successful development of a physical fitness program. This is especially true within the working environment where human interrelations, professional images, responsibilities and stresses are manifest. In such an environment emotional stakes are high and can become powerful defenders of the status quo. If the idea of a fitness program threatens any of these emotional stakes, active resistance may even ensue.

For example, the same aggressiveness and determination that made an executive a top manager may be responsible for his turning down an exercise plan because he once used these characteristics himself at an attempt to get into shape and failed. He may have then decided that if he couldn't do it, why should he pay for his underlings to fail as well.

The answer to this problem is to analyze this individual's attempt and determine the shortcomings of his or her original fitness plan. Once the manager understands the reason for the failure in terms that do not challenge his or her own characteristics, a new attempt at a personal fitness plan can be suggested. Once a program works for a manager there is a good likelihood that he or she will approve an employee fitness program based on the same principles.

Another barrier results from the manager who is himself unfit and has not been motivated to exercise or modify his lifestyle. This person does not want to involve himself in organizing a program for his employees. Most of the solutions to this problem have to do with motivating the manager and will be discussed in a later section dealing with motivation. However, in some instances such a person may see a company program as a personal opportunity for fitness. In other cases a superior or a board of directors could mandate that a manager seriously look into the development of a fitness program.

It is also important to appreciate that individual managers may hesitate to endorse an employee fitness program without the support of all the department heads and executives. In a large organization leadership initiative should be solicited by first polling those executives more likely to acknowledge support of a program independent of peer support.

Another managerial barrier that should be recognized has to do with a manager's unwillingness to admit that he is not aware of the need for an employee fitness program. In fact, many managers and administrators spend as little as ten percent of their time working with internal matters and the remaining time negotiating or working with external organizations. Since role conflict in management can be a sensitive issue, any attempt to suggest that he or she has not considered the matter fully should be handled carefully.

Human nature presents similar obstacles in motivating employees to accept the idea of participating in a physical fitness program. A common attitude that is a barrier to health improvement programs is the "provider ethic." This ethic is the belief that if an individual is providing basic needs for his family he is healthy enough. A suggestion by an employer that he or she become healthier may seem an insult.

The "provider ethic" has a strong hold on many American workers. A worker may have many health problems. He or she may drink heavily to suppress somatic or psychological distress, or exhibit many risk factors for heart disease or cancer. But this person would reject an accusation of poor health, either direct or indirect, on the basis that he or she is a successful wage earner and thus a healthy member of society.

Once again the best way to overcome such barriers is with education, diplomacy, and the revealing of a sincere commitment to the employee's welfare. It should be noted that one of the things in favor of fitness program promotion is public awareness of the fitness revolution. A Lou Harris poll in 1978 confirmed that most people believe that health maintenance is the best way of curbing health care costs. There was an overwhelming support of public and employee fitness programs. Sixty percent of the respondents did not consider it an invasion of privacy if employers encouraged them to live healthier lives and attempted to help them do so.

Such information is in sharp contrast to debates over health care programs by public, business, and labor leaders, but it is one of the few things about which many people are in agreement. When programs for fitness become a real possibility at one's own workplace, however, the prospect can stimulate many facets of human nature that might be antagonistic. And there is still the forty percent who consider such programs an invasion of privacy!

Thus individual psychological defenses within the work environment should be viewed as potential obstacles to fitness program development. Individual sensitivities regarding competition, a threat to security or ego, or being "told" to exercise can be significant variables that dictate the potential success of a program.

Furthermore, these barriers are apparent within management and among the work force. It is important to note that such sensitivities are often supported by labor unions. No smoking rules, incentives and penalties for exercise, and other operations can be attacked by labor as a threat to job security.

The way to overcome these barriers is through a gradual policy of education, a supportive environment, and a sincere and visible commitment by top management.

The Time Barrier

Another common excuse for not supporting an employee fitness program is that there is just not enough time for such a program. Some employers may feel that there is not enough time to meet current deadlines, let alone time enough for employees to participate in exercise programs. In terms of the long run payoff such excuses obviously cannot be justified, but even in the short term the objection can be overruled.

R. H. Dobbs, Jr., president of the Life Insurance Company of Georgia, counters the argument this way. "Our people do participate in our physical fitness program. And on company time. In fact, I insist on it. If they can't leave their jobs for at least one hour, two or three times a week, they're not organized and they shouldn't be in an executive position!"

Mr. Dobbs' statement is both justifiable and responsible. Furthermore, the argument is applicable not only to top executives but to most employees. Industry pays when employees lack enthusiasm, are bored with a routine, and want to call it a day two hours before quitting time. Any program that would help eliminate such work delays would automatically increase work time, not diminish it.

The adage, "If you want to get something done, give it to a busy man" is definitely applicable to the time barrier to becoming physically fit. If a person is organized, efficient, and motivated to carry out responsibilities, the additional responsibility of participating in a physical fitness program can be handled in stride. A good example is former President Jimmy Carter, who adheres to one of the busiest schedules in the country. Since undertaking his own running program during his tenure in the White House, he managed to lower his resting pulse rate from sixty to forty beats a minute, maintained a blood pressure of 120/80, and trimmed nine pounds. However history may view his accomplishments, he has managed to keep both his appointments and his health in that stressful position.

The Medical Menace

Industrial medical departments and physicians have an important role to play in determining the success of a fitness program. Emotionalism about physical fitness programs is prevalent among such medical personnel. Emotional stakes in a profession that may seem threatened by prevention programs can bring about the same defense mechanisms as those discussed previously. An individual in charge of the health of employees may know little about physical fitness, lifestyle, and nutrition, and may be hesitant to support a fitness plan.

At any rate, the medical department can make or break a fitness program. If the medical personnel are sincerely concerned about the well-being of the employee, educated beyond the scope of their medical school and internship, and energetic in their duties, powerful support can be expected. If however the medical director retired to the position to get away from a busy pediatric practice and other problems, a hard well can be expected.

An unsupportive medical department can be considered a major obstacle to the development of a fitness program. Employers have too much faith in medical services. Because of third party payment systems, most employers have no idea what kind of medical costs the company is absorbing. They really don't know what they are paying for because of their faith in the resident medical department.

For example, most companies started a physical exam schedule to protect their investment in employees. Standard physical exams rarely have any effect on the health of an employee. There is little evidence that the traditional annual physical can detect disease in its primary stages. Most diseases do not require a medical doctor to find. More than ninety percent of breast cancer, for example, is discovered by self-examination. Health screening, not disease screening, is what is effective.

Thus more education is in order. In the interim, however, there must be cooperation between upper management, the medical department, and personnel involved in promoting the physical fitness program. There must also be cooperation between the employees and the medical department. Employees should be confident that their medical records as well as their fitness records will be kept confidential and that the fitness program is totally supported by the company medical department. Information concerning medical prescription for exercise will be presented in Chapter 9.

It may be important to note that until people actually start enjoying the benefits of improved health and fitness, it may not be effective to educate participants too radically about the inadequacies of their faith in the traditional medical practice. Individuals may temporarily need the "hands on" effect that their faith in the medical profession provides. Seventy percent of the health problems seen at the Equitable Insurance Company Health Center, according to director Dr. Wolfsie, are psychosomatic. An attempt to educate these people about when to use the medical facility and when not to use it may be ineffective until the manifestations of poor health are actually relieved. And the fitness program will not be seen as a rival to the institution in which such a high trust is placed.

Most business organizations are influenced by a bureaucracy, both within and outside the organization. The bureaucratic system can be a barrier to fitness program implementation as it can be to any attempt at innovation in policy. A failure to recognize the limits and repercussions of bureaucracy, however, can cause business and industry to lose more than health care costs and productivity.

The inadequacies of a bureaucracy often result in the "red tape" syndrome. Red tape implies a lack of control. If people within an organization know what they are supposed to do they will do it and there will be no breakdown in communication, no lengthy delays, and no buck passing. But if the philosophy of work embraces a resistance to change and preset answers to unimagined problems, red tape is an inevitability.

Drucker says that the right way to define a problem so as to make it capable of resolution is to create, build, and maintain an attitude within the organization that sees change as a norm rather than an exception. This requires a certain restructuring of relations between top management and employees and will be in harmony with the ideal foundations for a successful fitness program.

Such an approach will not only minimize the bureaucratic barrier to fitness program implementation, it will also protect American business and industry from governmental controls that may eventually mean the decline and demise of the corporation.

This book's concern over government intervention into private industry is two-fold. First, since the factors that could be responsible for the corporate decline are similar to those responsible for inappropriate health care within business and industry, a mutual motive for improvements in health care exists. Secondly, if government intervention does increase to such a degree, it is unlikely that improvements in health care will actually occur.

A larger governmental role in regulating private safety and health care programs is not likely to be successful. The bureaucracy of government will be haphazardly lax in some areas and overzealous in others. It may just intensify current health care problems by mandating traditional modalities. The growth of governmental bureaucracies will frustrate attempts by private industry to reallocate resources and to shift health care planning to meaningful and economically productive enterprises, namely the implementation of health maintenance and physical fitness programs.

Since the goal of this book is improved health and fitness among Americans, it would be of no concern to its author whether it is private industry or government that accommodates appropriate action. However, the bureaucracy of government appears more inevitable than in business. Furthermore, governmental priorities are influenced by special interests, and as will be seen in later chapters, the health of the American people is often for sale.

Also, governmental regulations aimed at providing health and safety have not been too successful. Intervention by the FDA into control of chemicals has been suffocatingly slow. The Occupational Safety and Health Administration has been largely ineffective. Practically no one in the organization is trained to study, recognize, or treat occupational disease. There is almost no enforcement of its guarantees to a safe and healthful workplace with only five hundred inspectors for over four million workplaces. In one bill, lobbyists managed to eliminate five out of six workplaces from the laws; of millions of dollars in fines, only a small percentage have been collected.

Thus it can be seen that the elimination of bureaucratic inefficiencies within an organization can protect both the organization and the health of its employees from the inefficiencies of the bureaucracies outside of the organization. Business leaders must restructure organizational attitudes that reflect a concern for social welfare and employee health. A 1979 Gallup poll showed a tremendous need for business and industry to improve public relations. Businesses are for the most part distrusted. Such an environment can put private business in a precarious political position and can put fitness programs for the American worker back many years.

Legal Considerations

According to Dr. Martin L. Collis, author of the Canadian pamphlet on "Employee Fitness," there are no legal obstacles in the way of the development of an employee fitness program. Similarly, the President's Council on Physical Fitness and Sports published the following in their manual on "Physical Fitness in Business and Industry:"

"Safety and liability are two common objections to a fitness facility. Neither one will withstand serious scrutiny, and employee fitness facilities, like office parties or picnics, necessarily expose companies to some liability. These risks should be fully protected by liability insurance or a workmen's compensation plan."

Although any company launching such a program should examine its insurance policy or compensation act carefully and obtain additional coverage if necessary, the consensus of legal opinion is that if a program is properly organized and has normal liability insurance, legal problems should not be a barrier.

In spite of these observations, the worry over legal implications remains one of the most common objections to program implementation. The possibility of a lawsuit, however, is quite remote if the following guidelines are used in establishing the fitness program.

1. A complete medical questionnaire is a liability safeguard. If someone would die in an exercise session, the questionnaire might indicate a medical cause to the problem that was pre-existing. In many situations, however, such a questionnaire is neither practical nor accurate. Instead, use of the PAR Q and PAR X questionnaires, developed and approved by the Canadian government, should suffice. The former is provided for duplication in the Appendix.

2. Individuals who should not participate in the program without a written recommendation from a physician (or completion of PAR X) include anyone having a positive response on the PAR Q, anyone with a resting, sitting blood pressure of 150/100 or higher, or anyone with a resting pulse rate of 100 or higher.

3. An informed consent documentation should be signed by all participants for both testing and program participation. Sample forms are included in the Appendix. (Negligence is *not* avoided by an informed consent.)

4. Personnel who conduct testing and exercise programs should be certified in emergency care and cardio-pulmonary resuscitation. They should also have a thorough knowledge of the danger signs and symptoms which signify that testing or exercise should terminate or slow down. Some insurance policies require use of a certified fitness specialist.

5. Exercise prescription should be in accordance with the results of the tests or fitness evaluations (see Chapter 9).

6. Fitness leaders should limit their advice to their area of expertise and should not try to "practice medicine."

7. The testing and exercise facilities should be in good order and safe with no dangerous projections, weaknesses, floor irregularities, or other hazards.

If the above guidelines are followed, it is more likely that a lawsuit or grievance will result from ancillary policies than from accidents or injuries resulting from the actual exercise. For example, incentives for participation, smoking prohibition, or physical fitness standards may be considered discriminatory by certain individuals or unions.

But if the program is organized according to the philosophies of this book such reactions will be rare. The Sentry Insurance Company's physical fitness policy even extends into their hiring practice. They will not hire employees who smoke, drink excessively, or would not be willing to exercise regularly. According to the program director, Dr. D. Johnson, "We are willing to go to court over this policy."

Failure to endorse a fitness program because of legal considerations is more apt to be an excuse than a reason. In such cases it may be worth pointing out that there may be a higher liability lawsuit risk to an organization to leave employees out of a fitness program. Insurance companies and liability law consider that certain risks exist in business because a firm is legally responsible for employee activities. Considering that the majority of American business is service oriented, there are many opportunities for negligent and hazardous service resulting from inadequate coordination, heart attack, poor reaction time, or other consequences of poor health and fitness.

Speaking of legal liability in the context of employee fitness, the renowned exercise physiologist Dr. P. O. Astrand stated, "The most interesting lawsuit will come from someone who has a heart attack in his office and sues the company for forcing him to work in sedentary and stressful circumstances for many years." Considering the fact that industrial accidents represent a very small percentage of medical liability claims compared to on-the-job heart attacks, such a suit should demand more attention than those that might result from participation in a fitness program.

Decision Making

In the final analysis, the only real barriers to an employee fitness program are impairments to sound decision making in general. In view of the facts about improved health and fitness via employee fitness programs, failure to develop a program will probably reflect management's unwillingness to make a decision, a premature or snap decision, confusion over information, fear of mistakes, ignorance of the problem, or an emotional bias.

It is not that making corporate policy decisions is an easy task.

There are many external and internal pressures with which to contend. Economic conditions, conflicting value systems, available information, and self-interest groups must be faced. But if management can efficiently identify the objectives, rate the risks, and identify and evaluate the various alternatives, implementation of some type of fitness program will surely meet with some success.

At a meeting in the Roosevelt room in the White House, President Carter met with the President's Council on Physical Fitness and Sports about American employee fitness programs. During the discussion he spoke of the highly advanced employee fitness programs in Japan and pointed to the fact that they lead the world in both longevity and in productivity. He also mentioned that the programs were well received by management and were implemented accordingly. And he expressed hope that a similar phenomenon would overcome all the barriers to successful employee fitness programs in this country.

SNJ-MED-66-2A
FITNESS PROGRAM RECORD

NAME

SOCIAL SECURITY NO.	REPORT DATE MM DD YY	COMPANY	BIRTH DATE MM DD YY	SEX (M = 1, F = 2)	F - 1 NF = 2 P = 2	CODE	STATUS

PHYSICAL EXAMINATION

TEST TYPE (1 = STRESS, 2 = FOLLOW UP)

	BLOOD PRESSURE	PULSE	EKG
SUPINE-BASELINE	/		
STANDING-BASELINE	/		
EXERCISING AT TARGET	/		
(6MIN SUPINE) RECOVERY-POST EXERCISE	/		

COMMENTS:
GENERAL
LUNGS
HEART

STRESS TEST

MAXIMUM GRADE	
MAXIMUM SPEED	
TIME TO REACH TARGET (MINUTES)	
DISTANCE (REVOLUTIONS)	
COMMENTS:	

LABORATORY DATA

HEMOGLOBIN (g/100 ml)
ERYTHROCYTES (million/cu mm)
HEMATOCRIT (ml/100 ml)
CHOLESTEROL -FASTING (mg/100 ml)
TRIGLYCERIDE-FASTING (mg/100 ml)
GLUCOSE-FASTING (mg 100 ml)
URIC ACID-FASTING (mg/100 ml)

CHEST X-RAY (CODED)	HEART
	LUNGS
PULMONARY FUNCTION	VITAL CAPACITY (as % of predicted)
	FEV 1.0%

CLEARANCE

CLEARANCE CODES   CODE

STATEMENT

1. FULL PARTICIPATION
2. PARTICIPATION NOT RECOMMENDED
3. PARTICIPATION NOT RECOMMENDED AT THIS TIME
4. LIMITED PARTICIPATION

COMMENTS AND OR RESTRICTIONS:

EXAMINING PHYSICIAN   CODE

FINAL CLEARANCE

ANTHROPOMETRIC MEASUREMENTS

DOMINANCE (1 = RIGHT, 2 = LEFT)

GRIP TESTS (LBS)	RIGHT HAND	
	LEFT HAND	
SKIN FOLD MEASUREMENTS (MM)	TRICEPS	
	SUBSCAPULAR	
	ABDOMEN	
	THIGH	
BODY MEASUREMENTS (INS.)	CHEST - INSP.	
	CHEST - EXP.	
	ABDOMEN RELAXED	
HEIGHT	(INCHES)	
WEIGHT	AT PRESENT	
	AT AGE 21	
	MINIMUM SINCE 21	
	MAXIMUM SINCE 21	

BICYCLE ERGOMETRY	KPM/MIN.	
	TIME (SECONDS)	
	PULSE RATE	

SMOKING & COFFEE HISTORY	NOW SMOKING CIGARETTES/DAY	
	YEARS OF CIGARETTE SMOKING	
	YEAR DISCONTINUED 19	
	PACK YEARS	
	NOW DRINKING COFFEE - CUPS DAY	

ACTIVITY MNEMONIC	CODE	HRS.	YRS.

SUBJECTIVE RATINGS	BODY IMAGE	
	PRESENT ACTIVITY	
	PRESENT FITNESS	

FITNESS VERFICATION   CODE

A Typical Fitness Program

5

PROGRAM PROMOTION

A fitness program that is to include a significant portion of employees who are in need of it will not happen by itself. Spontaneous programs initiated by small groups of employees usually result in fit people keeping other fit people fit. If a productive fitness program is to be developed it will require a major selling campaign. This will be true whether it is being promoted by management, sub-management, or an outside fitness facility. Everyone who will have anything to do with the program must be involved in making the decision. The concept must be sold before a decision is made.

An effective decision to implement a fitness program is a commitment to action and results. Too many physical fitness programs have started and failed because of inadequate salesmanship. Enthusiasm in developing a fitness program can often be responsible for disregarding many important aspects of program organization. Patience may be difficult for the anarchist, but it is essential. E. A. Emmick, manager of Employee Services for North American Rockwell Corporation of El Segundo, California, and Ken White, Personnel Representative, spent seven years doing public relations work within their company before their successful program was implemented.

As a result of such efforts, the environment is becoming more conducive to the acceptance of fitness programs. Fitness is becoming an ideal product to sell for many reasons. Large numbers of populations are becoming receptive to the notion that self-responsibility is the key to wellness. It is more costly than ever to become sick. The anti-smoking movement is catching on. The women's movement is emphasizing fitness as is the advertising media. Research on the benefits of exercise is being published more often. There is a growing number of physicians who are becoming regular exercisers, and there is an increase in the number of companies that have fitness programs.

Such outside influences are important but it is especially helpful if receptivity is high within the company. Robert Silket, vice president of General Foods, states it bluntly; "We have a fitness program because the chairman of the board is an exercise enthusiast!" There are more and more company presidents, board directors, and stockholders who are personally involved in the fitness quest.

There are other determinants that increase fitness program feasibility inside the company. A reasonably good profit picture during the previous year may increase the chance of program approval. It is also helpful if there is at least one senior manager whose schedule will permit a certain amount of availability to implement a program. A medical department or director who is interested in a fitness program will enhance the chances of successes significantly. And a high level of employee morale and good relations between management and employees may be contributory.

Frequently all of these conditions will not exist. At any rate a fitness program promoter is invariably going to meet with some sharp resistance at the outset. It is imperative that effective salesmanship be practiced at the very beginning.

The Committee

The first step in selling a fitness program to an organization is to start the formation of a planning and research committee. If the promotion is not initiated by company management, an official sanction should be requested for the development of a "health care cost containment" committee. This request should be developed informally by individuals concerned with both the well-being of the company employees and the high costs of health care within the company and the community. If the actions of the committee do not require a significant amount of company time it is unlikely that the request will be turned down.

Once sanction has been granted, the formation of the committee should be announced to all members of the organization. Everyone interested should be given an opportunity to be appointed and those not selected to serve should be placed in an advisory capacity. It is very important, however, that the committee include representatives from upper management, occupational health, personnel, employee groups, and labor unions. Without powerful representation the conclusions of the committee will receive lower priority than other projects staffed by higher level personnel.

The formation of a committee called something like "health care cost containment" will avoid any initial reaction to the more specific objective, i.e. a fitness program. Indeed the committee should be unbiased in its analysis and various alternatives should be considered including blood pressure screening programs, health education bulletins, or diet reduction and smoking education pamphlets and seminars. The conclusion that a total fitness program would be the most effective means of improving health and containing costs should be approached and reported as a logical deduction.

Once the committee is formed, its first function should be to acquire information regarding the company's medical costs and history of disabilities, absenteeism, and premature retirements. This information can be used to illustrate the need for some action.

The second step should be to prepare a questionnaire describing the needs and health problems in the company and presenting several alternative solutions. Each solution should be described with regard to its implementation feasibility and the benefits that could be expected. This questionnaire may establish a desire on the part of management and employees for a fitness program. To accomplish this it is important that the questionnaire is titled or introduced so as to show it originated from the committee and not from management. The questionnaire will also help determine the potential participation level that can be expected in the fitness program.

Management Initiated Programs

If the desire for a fitness program originates from top management, it is especially important that the committee and the questionnaire appear responsive as opposed to paternalistic. Otherwise the entire subject of health care innovation may become threatening to employees. After the questionnaires are completed and collected the concerned manager should then begin an informal campaign to educate all managers, sub-managers, and employees about the conclusions. Films, lectures, button-holing, and lunch conversations should all be aimed at opening up channels of communication to establish a proper foundation for the program and stimulate a positive attitude.

The manager should realize that a failure to include all participants in the decision making in some way will contribute to the eventual failure of the program. He should see about selling the program to his employees and sub-managers as if they were customers of the business. If the program is implemented as an independent order from the top, retaliation can be expected from the lower ranks. Even with the power capabilities of demotion, salary cuts, or loss of job a top manager who wants a healthy, happy company cannot afford such tactics. Between the resentment stimulated and the retaliation of union groups, a successful program would have no chance.

Once the manager has stimulated a positive attitude about the fitness program concept, he should go back to the committee and have them prepare a specific needs analysis relating to fitness program feasibility. (This topic will be discussed in the next chapter.) When the specific program is recommended by the committee, an announcement can be made that the decision has been made to implement an employee fitness program for all personnel.

Labor Groups

One exception to the timeliness of the decision announcement is if the manager wants to use the fitness program as a collective bargaining item. If the interest in a fitness program is high among the employees a manager might want to offer the fitness program as a benefit to employees. In this case, the manager should muffle his own interest in a program and sell the idea to employees with a reverse psychology. Such is the game of collective bargaining.

In order for this approach to work there must be a very high interest level among employees for a fitness program and it must be presented in an attractive package, usually giving company time for exercise. Otherwise most employee groups and unions may turn down an offer in lieu of more immediate monetary benefits.

The use of physical fitness programs as a collective bargaining item is a tricky issue. This is because fitness programs are both an investment and a benefit. The company is investing in increased productivity and decreased medical costs while the employee is benefiting from improved health and job satisfaction. When Janet Redick turned a job offer down with one company to join Northern Natural Gas Company in Omaha, Northern Gas benefited. But because she turned down the other offer so she could enjoy Northern's fitness program and facility, she made the decision because of a personal benefit.

Looking at it from the other side of the table, an article in *Nation's Business* illustrated future collective bargaining possibilities based on the enjoyment of fitness programs by employees. The article opens with the hypothetical conversation:

"The tough union negotiator took a long look at the proposed health insurance package that his company counterpart, with a wince at its cost, had just laid on the table."

"Forget that," the union man said. "What kind of physical fitness facilities can you provide?"

Sub-Management Initiated Programs

The same reverse psychology in collective bargaining can be used by employee groups or unions who want a physical fitness program. This is a bit remote but it is possible that an employee group could offer to establish and participate as a group in a fitness program in trade for a wage increase or other benefit. This, of course, would only work if management was educated and convinced that such a program would indeed decrease operating costs and disabilities and increase productivity. And it would be essential that a high percentage of employees were contractually guaranteed to participate regularly in the program.

In most cases a sub-management initiated fitness program will be aimed at management's implementation of a program. After the concerned employee has organized an officially sanctioned "health cost containment" committee and questionnaires have been completed by all members of the organization, a specific needs analysis of fitness program implementation should be accomplished and informal campaigning should begin.

Although it may seem more appropriate for sub-management to seek approval more formally through official type communication channels, such channels make immediate rejection too simple. Again, everyone must have an opportunity to be involved in deciding to have a fitness program before it is actually sold to the decision maker. This is not democracy, it is good salesmanship. People are less likely to abuse an innovation if they were involved in its implementation.

Another reason for the informal initial approach is that it represents the first attempt at breaking down the bureaucratic barriers. The impersonality of such barriers may currently guide the activities of the company, but will stifle the promotional and motivational efforts necessary for a successful fitness program. It should be realized that the informal campaign is not an attempt to totally change the system, but merely to set a proper stage for the fitness innovation.

Another reason the informal approach is appropriate is because top management personnel know that decisions must first be based on opinions, then facts. A corporate leader wants to know the relevance of events to his or her business. He is somewhat distrustful of statistics because he knows a good statistician can find facts to support almost any conclusion. An effective executive is concerned with understanding as well as facts, and such understanding is best facilitated by open, informal communication among many speakers.

Once education and response has been initiated via the question-naire and the informal campaigning, and a formal, objective, specific needs plan has been drawn by the committee, the next step is to decide who is the ultimate decision maker. In many cases it will be the same authority that sanctioned the formation of the commit-tee. In some situations the plan may have to go through a chain of command before it reaches the ultimate decision maker, but it is essential that the plan does not dead end along the way. A proper pre-plan campaign and a good presentation combined with the fact that the committee is comprised of formidable individuals will assure that the proposal will at least keep moving, regardless of the recommendations of a particular link in the chain.

In many cases it may be preferable to pass the plan through vari-ous department heads for their endorsement. If it is likely that positive recommendations will be made, the plan will be all the more appealing to the final decision maker, whether it be a board or an individual. For some companies the final decision makers may exist in an entirely different locale, and such endorsements may be extremely helpful.

Sometimes it will be difficult to determine exactly who has the final decision making authority. A business may not have clearly defined authority for making decisions about innovations. In such businesses authority has been designated only within the confine-ments of defined regulations. If such a "catch 22" situation does exist, it may be impossible to contact a group of scattered, disinter-ested stockholders who have failed to set up a procedure for innova-tive management. In such a case all that is required to implement a low-risk fitness program is an independent endorsement by who-ever is considered the "boss."

The final presentation to the decision maker can be made col-lectively by the committee members or individually by a charismatic individual who has emerged as a "champion" of the project. In either case, rational approaches to convincing or changing attitudes based strictly on data, analysis, and options are rarely enough to induce the change. Instead, psychological approaches may be necessary.

In understanding what approach to use, the style of leadership and decision making processes should be analyzed and the presen-tation should be emphasized accordingly. A primary objective of the "salesman" should be to determine the decision maker's mana-gerial philosophy as categorized by Blake, Mouton, and Foss. Blake and Mouton described two managerial theories of motivation that included a concern for production and a concern for people. Foss later added a third theory which represented a concern for a company as a sub-system of a larger social system. According to the theories, every manager has a philosophy that ranges somewhere between the three.

If such a style can be ascertained, the sales presentation should be aimed at the particular viewpoint. If the concern is primarily for production, then the emphasis should be on the advantages of a fitness program to company productivity. If the more obvious concern is for the employees, the emphasis should be on the increased well-being resulting from a fitness program. If the manager's philosophy emphasizes the social responsibility of the company, then the national ramifications of the employee fitness program should be most pronounced.

Other particular interests and philosophies can be observed besides the above. For example, the president of a company in Spokane had attempted for several years to set up programs that gave the workers more responsibility. He wanted them to start setting objectives based on their own knowledge of productivity as opposed to the traditional procedures. The programs he wanted to implement proved to be too much of a risk and never became a reality.

When an employee group presented a proposal for an employee fitness program, they emphasized that it would be an excellent way to see if employees could set and proceed with independent objectives without risking production objectives. The employees had done their homework. The company now has a fine fitness facility.

There are many other psychological considerations regarding the personality, interests, and style of leadership of the manager. An obvious example would be if the manager was a post-coronary patient. Then the fitness program emphasis could be on how many heart attack victims have successfully run marathons after participating in a company fitness program. Such specifics only need be determined by someone who is perceptive and has known the individual well.

The psychological approach is effective not only in the formal presentation to the decision maker, but in informal presentations to managers, sub-managers, and members of the committee who may not be convinced of the role an employee fitness program might play in containing costs and increasing productivity. One psychological approach that is successful in the informal situation is to first work on an element that a person only mildly disagrees with, then gradually working on the whole. This approach recognizes that the greater the obvious pressure in trying to convince someone the more likely the resistance. Persuasion works best when a person is unaware it is happening.

One example of indirect persuasion applicable to selling fitness concepts is referred to by Varela as "successive approximation and reactance." First of all, the goal should be kept in mind, i.e., the implementation of a physical fitness program. The immediate objective is to stimulate a personal commitment to the idea of a fitness program via a *series of gradual affirmations*. As in the formal presentation, enough research should be done to know a little about the target's personality, concerns, values, and philosophies. Considering human nature and the unique sensitivities that prevail regarding physical fitness, such methodologies are appropriate in the attempt to sell a fitness program to top management.

Causing changes in attitudes and organizations is a major challenge to whoever is willing to put himself on the line to challenge the status quo. Drucker says that making innovative organizations the rule in America, rather than the exception, is still largely an unsolved task. Perhaps one solution is simple salesmanship combined with courage to take the initiative for innovative proposals that challenge the status quo.

If every attempt to develop a fitness program in a company fails, there is a last resort, if the fitness program is important enough for its champion to risk his job. If management absolutely refuses to make any concessions toward giving employees an opportunity for fitness, public pressure and employee group pressure might be brought to bear on the organization. This would require the willingness of the media to support the attack on management's unwillingness and would require the organization of labor against management's stand on the issue.

Outside Initiated Programs

The near future will see the development of a new type of business, an employee fitness service. Although there are already several in existence, the need for such services will lead to an increase in the number. In the Blue Cross manual, "Building a Healthier Company," the fact that a company is pretty much on its own is emphasized sized several times. "Unfortunately, company involvement in employee/executive fitness programs has grown so fast that it has outrun manpower and information resources."

If an individual wishes to begin such a business, he should first become a qualified fitness specialist or acquire a staff so trained. Equally important is the availability of a good salesman.

The next step is to search for companies that might be especially receptive to the idea of implementing a fitness program. Such companies might include those planning new facilities, companies that have facilities already present for staff recreational use, companies with a known interest in fitness, and companies that have an obvious investment in their personnel or a high rate of disability and turnover.

Once target companies have been selected, it is recommended that informal marketing techniques be employed in the community where the business is located. This can be done through writing articles for newspapers, magazines, inter-office newsletters, and speaking at local organization meetings. Other methods are through informing board members, committee members, and other community members about the service being for sale to companies.

After the informal techniques have been implemented, the seller should send a brochure to all possible companies that have been targeted explaining the highlights of the service offered. This should be followed up by a letter addressed to a person in the company who is a key figure in the decision making process or who is highly influential on the decision maker. This individual might be on the Board of Managers, or a medical director, or the company recreational director, a vice-president, or the president. It is important, however, that the individual have direct communication with top management.

An appointment should then be made with a decision maker in the company. If possible a physician or someone within the company who can act as a liason should accompany the seller at the meeting. The presentation needs to have a graphic picture of the program that is being sold. This picture, however, can only be partial as a specific needs analysis will have to be done within the company to determine the unique needs and resources of the company. The first objective is to receive a contract that will allow the seller to implement this analysis. There should be a cost attached to the analysis that is deductible from the program cost if a decision is made to implement a program.

After the specific needs analysis is completed (see next chapter), a second appointment should be scheduled with the decision maker for the final sale. At this meeting the entire program should be outined along with specific measurable goals and objectives.

Once a program is sold, the fitness service must then commence with implementing it. Program implementation will be discussed in Chapter 8.

For those companies interested in contacting a fitness service that is already in operation, the following organizations may be of help.

The President's Council on Physical Fitness and Sports can send information and recommend some area services, and the American Association of Fitness Directors in Business and Industry has a published list of regional contacts that may be of assistance. This list is included in the Appendix.

There are also several fitness services already established on the West Coast including Motivational Fitness Seminars in Novato, California, Fitness Systems, Inc. in Los Angeles, Fitness Motivation Institute in Palo Alto, California, the California Health Research Foundation, Kentfield, California, the Corporate Cup Association in Mountain View, California, Karagama and Associates, Saugus, California, Risk and Claims Ltd., San Francisco, California, Fitness Resources, Menlo Park, California, and Motivational Fitness Assessment and Seminars, Mann County, California. There are also many Y.M.C.A. organizations that are providing employee fitness service.

6

NOTING THE NEEDS

Making the best use of the resources available and applying them to the specific needs of the company is the first and most important step in implementing a successful fitness program. Determining these needs requires careful analysis of the many variables that can affect the success of the fitness program. These variables include:

- financial resources available for program
- space available for exercise, testing, and lectures
- number of potential participants
- characteristics and interests of prospective participants
- work and time schedules
- equipment needed for implementation
- educational program needs
- alternative fitness programs
- leadership
- testing protocols
- motivational considerations

In addition to the above, the analysis should also include specific data relating to the company's history of medical costs, premature retirement, and disability. It should be remembered that a concise report on the fitness needs and solutions will be presented to top management for the final decision to initiate program development.

Money

The amount of money a company is willing to invest in an employee fitness program is dependent on the expectations of a return on the money and actual funds available. A high combination of both might result in a fitness center that is spread over two thousand acres and includes a twelve thousand square foot double gym, a six thousand square foot single gym, a swimming pool, and playing fields that would be the envy of a major university. Xerox, for example, has such a facility. It cost about two million dollars and is used by over fifteen hundred trainees and staff.

Obviously not every company will have such ample funds available nor will every company have the confidence in the investment to warrant too large an expenditure. In any case, programs can be proposed to satisfy management. Unless the seller-promoter knows beforehand the exact level of confidence and money available, it is recommended that two or three alternative programs be designed to accommodate the situation. The most ideal program, in terms of a success ratio for a large number of employees, should be presented first. The second and third alternatives should require a less significant investment in terms of time or money.

For the company that is reluctant to make a large commitment to an employee fitness program for fear of program failure, it may be helpful to inform management that a program can be implemented that is not a long-term commitment and that can be reversed or abandoned without a significant loss of production. It should further be pointed out that there would be no negative impact on other functions and areas of the business. In addressing these two concerns the seller will be displaying an appreciation of the characteristics that determine the nature of a business decision about which there is some doubt.

Such considerations can be appreciated, but not emphasized. In the final analysis the budget proposal will be a reflection of the value of the program. The value of the program will be based on the company's problems that can be related to poor fitness compared to the calculated effect of the fitness program on an estimated number of regular participants. Within the limits of actual available money, this should be the ultimate criterion.

If the company is hesitant in initiating a full-scale program, it may consider implementing a small-scale program for a select population of employees. In most instances the select population are the executive level employees. It is preferable, however, if a mixed population of employees is used for the "experiment." In this way a more accurate assessment can be made of the potential success of a large-scale program.

This approach can also be used as a long-term developmental concept. The program can be designed so as to remain limited to a small number of personnel. Attendance records can be kept on participants and those not regularly making use of the program can be ousted to make room for the next employee on a waiting list. This type of program is used successfully by several companies. Gradually, if the waiting list, facilities, and financial resources warrant it, the program can be enlarged to include more employees.

Another low-budget alternative is to develop a "ground floor" fitness program initially. This type of program requires only a professional fitness specialist. There is no need for a capital expenditure for equipment or facilities and the only costs are those attributable to retaining such an individual.

The "ground floor" fitness program is an educationally based program with a minimum of motivational aspects. The objectives of such a program are to increase the knowledge of fitness among employees and to show how fitness can have a personal meaning for employees. The essence of the program involves the specialist's involvement in circulating educational material and organizing lectures. It also involves soliciting people to participate in informal group exercise programs during lunch breaks, before and after work and in some cases during the work day.

One such program has been implemented successfully at the Bankers' Life & Casualty Company in Chicago. At 4:30 p.m., about forty employees cross the street to a community center with gym clothes in hand. By five o'clock, fitness instructor Tom Gulan starts the exercise class. In an interview with Chicago correspondent Marcia Opp, he stated that he can conduct classes in any building as long as he has a stopwatch. "Fancy equipment is not needed to keep people fit and happy," he said.

Although any program can be started like this, its success as a permanent type of program is largely dependent upon a significant number of employees who are highly receptive to the idea of employee exercise programs. This can be determined with questionnaires and interviews during the specific needs analysis. The success of this type of program is also highly influenced by the quality of the chosen fitness specialist.

A second type of program that requires a slightly higher investment in terms of facilities incorporates fitness testing for each employee. This will require a minimal capital expenditure, depending on the sophistication of the testing equipment, for the equipment and additional costs for recordkeeping and time costs for the specialist. Testing will be discussed in detail in Chapter 10, but it should be noted here that the additional expense of testing in terms of attracting and keeping more participants is well worth the investment.

With no more than the above described facilities, many companies have developed highly successful fitness programs. Walking and or running programs during the noon hour are commonplace among such companies as Memorex, ESL Inc., National Semiconductor Corporation, Fairchild, Teledyne, Hewlett-Packard and many others. Other companies, especially those located in inclement environments, have programs of exercise in basements, on rooftops, and in empty lecture rooms. Although they have plans for a new facility, Metropolitan Life has had a program whereby employees simply run through the corridors and up and down stairways. Other companies have made exercise circuits in their corridors by simply designing various exercise stations along the route.

Another idea that has been implemented successfully in several companies is the charging of employees for participation in the program. This approach might be used by a company that is willing to make an initial capital investment but wants to reduce the risk and costs of operation. The decision to use this approach should be based on questions devised in a survey and the costs to an employee should be modest. In most cases the financing of a fitness center is split between the company and the staff.

At Weyerhaeuser in Tacoma, Washington, for example, the operation is on a club basis, with a subscription fee of nine dollars and fifty cents a month. Total membership in the club is well over three hundred and the facilities are steadily expanding. Administration of the club is in the hands of a board of trustees, elected by the members themselves.

At the General Foods Fitness Center there is an annual charge of fifty dollars per participating employee. The fee is deducted from the payroll. The second year of its existence, membership in the fitness program increased one hundred percent and in 1978 almost one-third of the three thousand employees had signed up.

The Michigan Department of Public Health implemented a program with the approval of Governor William Milliken that charged the participants for each segment of the program. Individual fitness testing was done on an individual fee basis, as was exercise counseling. At Xerox, any employee, his family, and retirees are eligible to take part in their fitness program for nine dollars per year per person. At Batelle Memorial Institute in Columbus, Ohio, ten percent of twenty-five hundred employees pay a fee of three dollars a month for a program that includes use of the gymnasium, swimming pool, and various recreational and educational activities. At Georgia Life's Health and Fitness Club, annual implementation costs of seventy-five thousand dollars are assisted by charging their current membership of two hundred fifty six dollars per month per person.

Perhaps the least expensive commitment to an employee fitness program is exemplified by the "corporate subsidy program." In this program an employee brings verification that he or she is in a legitimate exercise program within the community. With proof of regular attendance of over fifty percent of the classes, the company will pay part of the price of the program. While such programs are indeed better than nothing at all, they leave much to be desired in terms of getting a significant percentage of employees fit.

With this last thought in mind, a New York Telephone Company executive once made an important statement relative to their own employee fitness program. He said, "New York Telephone wants evidence of cost effectiveness (of the fitness program) in terms of improving health, not dollars and cents!" This may be a more important concept for managers in considering their fitness programs.

Facilities

Successful fitness programs may not require costly facilities, but if money is available every attempt should be made to "buy" as much convenience as possible. The more convenient and accessible is a fitness facility the more long-term participants will use it. A facility that will regularly attract fewer than twenty-five percent of the employees of a company may not prove to be effective, efficient, or productive.

A fitness program with a circuit training room with showers, lockers, medical testing, individual exercise prescription, educational and motivational systems, and a full-time fitness staff can reach sixty to eighty percent of the marketplace. The incorporation of additional fitness alternatives inside and outside the company may have a potential impact on ninety percent of the employees. But even with these components and a significant financial investment, convenience is paramount to the achieving of such percentages.

Accessibility may be the difference between an employee choosing to remain in the cafeteria during lunch and choosing to exercise. For this reason it is preferable to develop the facility within the main building. If there is no space within the building, some companies have built a complete facility within a prefabricated trailer unit. If this alternative is used the trailer should be placed in as convenient a location from the building as possible. If space is leased nearby, the company should provide shuttle service during appropriate hours to and from the building that houses the facility.

Another factor is the existence of showers and lockers. A convenient place to change and a refreshing shower before returning to work often is a major determinant of whether or not a person chooses to participate in an exercise session. Ideally separate shower facilities for men and women should be built. If this is not possible, a shower room can be used on an alternating basis by men and women. If lockers cannot be placed in an area where clothes can be changed, the convenience of having a place to keep gym clothes is still worth having lockers somewhere in the building, even if changing must be done elsewhere.

As important as the shower facility may be, its existence should not be a contingency for participating in a fitness program. Many European employee fitness clubs operate with a significant number of participants without the amenities of showers and locker rooms. "Honest sweat has no odor," says Dr. George Sheehan, and a washing and toweling at a bathroom sink can prepare an individual for returning to work just about as well as a shower. A re-evaluation of values, being a part of a fitness program, may be necessary in many areas if the importance of exercise is going to outweigh more trivial priorities. Although a shower is an important convenience, it should not be a prerequisite.

The size of the fitness facility should be determined by the specific needs analysis. Surveys should be used to determine the potential number of participants and to determine at what time during the day they would use the facility. Once a fair estimate is made of peak use hours and the total number of participants that might be in the facility at one time, appropriate space can be considered to be about three square feet per person. This is especially applicable for group exercise activities, although a well-planned circuit training room might require less space.

The appearance of the facility is also of importance. Not only is an attractive exercise room conducive to participation but an attractive facility can be an asset to a company's recruitment program as well as its public relations program. An exercise room should be well ventilated but not drafty. It should be colorful and well lit. It should be noise insulated and it should be maintained immaculately.

Equipment

A successful fitness program may need no more than a room such as described above and a fitness leader. The specific needs analysis may indicate employees are more interested in the circuit training concept than a group exercise program. Usually both will be offered and individuals can choose between group sessions or individual circuit programs.

A circuit program facility is limited only by imagination, financial resources, and space. Circuits can be designed in corridors of buildings, in conference rooms, in specially built rooms and buildings, or outside of the building. A common circuit training concept is the Swiss designed "parcourse" that combines a jogging trail with various exercise stations that describe a specific exercise and number of repetitions to complete before continuing on to the next station. There are also many varieties of resistive weight circuit training equipment that can be purchased and housed in a small area.

An ideal circuit training program should begin with exercise stations that serve as a warm-up and end with stations that will serve as a cool-down. In this way exercise can begin and end gradually as it should. Competition between participants should be discouraged; rather, the exercises should be intra-personally competitive with the participant competing only with himself to achieve the goals set for him.

A good example of a circuit program is at Exxon's corporate headquarters building in Manhattan. The exercise room is a pleasant sunny area forty-six by twenty-eight feet with one wall of windows and two of mirrors, carpeted, with indirect lighting and central air conditioning. The room contains the following ten exercise stations which provide a good guideline for the types of alternatives that are desirable. A warm-up period of five minutes of stretching and calisthenics precedes the first station and follows the last station.

1. *Medicine ball throw* - A nine pound ball is thrown against a sensor pad mounted on the wall above head level. This builds up the extensor muscles of the arm and upper back and secondarily the flexors of the shoulder girdle as well as acting as a warm-up for the next station.

2. *Rope jump* (First cardiovascular stress) - The participant skips rope on a sensor pad for proper pacing. As in all the cardiovascular exercises, participants exercise according to the target heart rate as described in Chapter One.

3. *Wall-pulley weights* - This improves muscular strength, endurance and flexibility of the upper extremities, trunk, legs, and upper back. To some degree it prepares the participant for the next exercise.

4. *Rowing machine* (Second cardiovascular exercise) - In addition to the desired effect on the heart, the extensors and flexors of the

legs, the shoulder girdle, the extensors of the back, and the abdominal musculature are exercised.

5. *Knee-Thigh weights* - The quadriceps and hamstrings of the legs are strengthened and warmed up for the next station.

6. *Stationary bicycle ergometer* (Third cardiovascular stress) - The leg extensors are exercised, particularly the quadriceps in addition to the cardiovascular system.

7. *Sit-ups on a slant board with knees bent* - This exercise develops and maintains the strength and endurance of the abdominal musculature, aids in maintaining good posture and in the prevention of back problems.

8. *Treadmill* (Fourth cardiovascular stress) - This produces the greatest stress on the cardiovascular system as the participant runs on the treadmill at a designated speed and grade over a set distance.

9. *Dumbbells* (Cooling-down station) - This exercise improves the strength of the biceps and shoulder girdle and provides a cool-down for the treadmill.

10. *Punching bag* (Cooling-down station) - Eye-hand coordination is improved as well as the strength of the arm extensors.

The circuit concept of physical training accommodates a wide variety of schedules, produces an efficient means of optimal, properly directed exercises, and affords both individual and group participation. The variety of exercise stations and the short time at each one also reduces boredom fatigue often suffered when an entire session is done on one apparatus, e.g. an ergometer. Although a program should be devised based on the needs of the company, it should be noted that a group exercise program led by a qualified leader may hold the interest and improve the fitness of a larger number of participants. A third alternative that can be added is the addition of sports equipment.

The addition of sports and recreation equipment and facilities to a fitness program may reach those employees who are not attracted to either the circuit training or the group exercise training concept. Such equipment might include a basketball gym, gymnastic equipment, swimming pools, or handball courts. Although the distinction between recreational type activities and activities that produce target heart rate exercise must be remembered, proper directions for sports and recreational activities can produce effective exercise sessions. If proper exercise is accomplished, the relaxation and opportunity to play at recreational activities is an important adjunct to a fitness facility. A good example of an extensive fitness-recreational combination exists at the Sentry Insurance Company in Stevens Point, Wisconsin. Their fitness facility includes an Olympic size swimming pool, an exercise gym, a running track, a three-court gymnasium, handball courts, a theatre, and a restaurant.

resources with other companies to build fitness centers that are accessible to employees of all the companies. Investors building office buildings are adding multi-faceted fitness and recreation facilities to their complex and as a result are experiencing one hundred percent occupancy. Commercial enterprises are developing near business communities that offer a wide range of fitness facilities. In Manhattan a facility covers a full block and has eleven stories. It has eighteen tennis and squash courts, a six hundred foot running track, swimming pools, health club, dance floor, game rooms, and a restaurant.

Another commercial program offered amidst a number of corporations and business enterprises is "Physis." Located in an industrial center in downtown San Francisco, an eight hundred dollar investment will put an executive through a comprehensive three-month fitness program that includes medical screening, fitness testing and retesting, a directed cardiovascular exercise session, and a directed strength and flexibility session. The program is conducted in a beautiful, sophisticated setting with all the amenities including health foods and music.

The existence of such spas and fitness centers for businessmen attests to the interest of employee fitness programs and gives ample opportunity for businessmen to exercise. Such programs are not able to reach a high percentage of a company's employees however. It is for this reason that the same concepts used by such commercial enterprises should be adopted and built into a company's own organization when possible.

The variety and types of equipment that a facility should have are also largely determined by the unique characteristics of the employee population. These considerations also should determine the types of educational programs that will be offered. Various characteristics that might indicate specific equipment and programs include the average age and sex of the employees, how close to the facility most live, academic and athletic background of the majority, number of people that smoke or are significantly overweight, the aversion or inclination to competition of the average participant, and of course, the indicated interests of the population. An accurate assessment of these traits can be very helpful in building a facility that will be highly efficient.

Although women's liberation may have lessened the problem, the element of sex might offer some difficulties to a program. Many women and men are still self-conscious about their unfit appearance. Such individuals are unlikely to want to dress in gym clothes and exercise in front of members of the opposite sex. Although establishing separate schedules for males and females makes implementation more complicated, if the needs analysis and surveys indicate this preference, every attempt should be made to overcome such an excuse for not participating.

Scheduling

One of the most difficult needs to meet with a fitness program has to do with the work schedules of employees and the time allotted for exercise and program participation. One of the most important determinations is whether or not the facilities are to be available during the work hours. According to Duggar and Swengros little has been done in the history of employee fitness and recreation programs to provide exercise for employees during working hours. During the past decade, however, more and more companies are providing opportunities for employees to exercise during company time.

One of the major advantages of allowing employees to exercise on company time is that a larger number of participants will be drawn into the program. Even with a beautiful facility and adequate leadership, many individuals will not be motivated to come to work an hour early, stay an hour longer, or exercise during their lunch hour. Furthermore, as an employee realizes that he is actually getting paid to improve his or her fitness, an additional incentive exists to participate.

It should be noted that a joint statement of the President's Council on Physical Fitness and Sports and the American Medical Association's Committee on Exercise and Physical Fitness regarding guidelines for physical fitness programs in business and industry included the following recommendation: "At least a portion, if not all, of the physical fitness program should be conducted on company time for purposes of motivation and supervision. Many participants will engage in a prescribed program for a specified period of time and at the completion of that period, progress to other physical activities outside the company."

In most situations, group exercise programs may have to be reserved for before and after work and during lunch, and on-duty exercise will be done individually on a circuit, track, pool, etc. If a company is large enough and a work schedule permits larger numbers of employees to be away from their duties at one time, then an exception can be made. In any case, those employees who cannot leave their phone station, or assembly line position, or front desk duties, can often be relieved for an hour by someone else. The someone else might even be a top executive who hasn't worked in the lower ranks for years and would actually benefit the company by doing so!

For most occupations in the American service-oriented work force, employees should be able to organize their work schedule in such a way as to fit in the hour of exercise. It cannot be denied that most workers accumulate at least an hour's worth of coffee breaks and slowdowns to accommodate the time. And, as has been indicated, the vitality resulting from the program will provide more energy, stamina, and enthusiasm to carry out the day's duties.

There are many ways to handle the logistics of scheduling. Someday it may even seem important enough for employees to be fit that a company might close its doors to business an hour early so that everyone in the company might have the opportunity to participate. In some companies business can continue while employees don gym clothes and answer phones that might interrupt exercise or even greet customers in such attire, a new slant for public relations. A more conservative approach is to have various numbers of employees exercise on alternate work days, or perhaps letting employees off one-half hour early if they remain after work an additional one-half hour to complete the hour exercise program.

It has been suggested by some fitness directors that time for exercise be shared between employees and clients of a business as well. Such a unique idea has credibility in a business that attracts customers for longer periods of time. Instead of talking business over a martini, business transactions might be accomplished during a round of handball, running, or pushups. Such a program might also attract customers. An airport exercise facility, for example, might be a convenient place for a traveler to go before catching a flight. Or instead of waiting an hour in a dentist's office, a patient could wait and exercise at the same time.

Such suggestions might seem somewhat farfetched, but the opportunities for scheduling time to exercise require imagination as well as a commitment to the exercise priority. Furthermore, the positive attitudes of the public toward exercise might make such possibilities work very well.

HEALTH PRO MOTION PROGRAM PARAMETERS				
Type	Ease in Establishing Program	Frequency of Problem (High +++ Low +)	Relative Value of Intervention (High +++ Low +)	Relative Cost to Establish
Wiser Health Care Buyers	Easy	++	++	Low
First Aid/CPR	Easy	+	+	Low
Dental Hygiene	Easy	+	+	Low
Physical Fitness	Easy	+++	+++	Low
Nutrition and Obesity	Moderate	++	+	Low
Stress Reduction	Moderate	+	++	Low
Smoking Cessation	Moderate	+	++	Moderate
Alcohol/Chemical Abuse	Moderate	+++	+++	Moderate
High Blood Pressure	Moderate	+++	+++	Moderate

Behind the Scenes

To produce the optimal program, the specific needs analysis should spare no details. Very often the success of a program is dependent on the many details that might be overlooked. For example, if a large percentage of employees make use of a company cafeteria, there may be a need to modify the types and variety of foods offered. There may be a need to remove candy and cigarette machines from the building that should be addressed. If there is a significant problem with emotional disorders, a hypoglycemia education program might accompany the regular program. Similarly a significant number of heart attack victims might warrant a special post-coronary fitness program.

There are also many "behind the scenes" factors that are crucial to the success of a program. Record keeping, for example, is an extremely important consideration. Efficient records must be kept of attendance, fitness evaluations, and program evaluations. Continual education and motivation will require planning and efficient delivery. There may be a need for laundry service. Equipment should be kept in top working order. And scheduling plans and announcements should be continually updated.

Such needs will require manpower, and a company very often might have people available to handle these needs. Other alternatives include employees volunteering time and sharing tasks or the hiring of personnel. In any case, the needs and the possible solutions should be carefully considered at the outset of program development.

The most important needs of any fitness program are leadership and motivation. In the specific needs analysis, there may be motivational and leadership needs that are unique to a specific organization. Chapters seven and nine will address these needs.

7

THE LEADING ROLE

In most of the literature about fitness programs there is consistent agreement that leadership is the key to a successful fitness program. Dr. Richard Keelor of the President's Council on Physical Fitness has stated that "The key to a successful program is not facilities. It's leadership." Jim Witticker of the Life of Georgia concurs; "All that is needed (for a successful fitness program) is a shower room, a track, and a good, enthusiastic leader. If I had to give up anything I would give up the shower room first, the track second, and the leader last." A major study of fitness and recreation programs in Manitoba, Canada concluded similarly: "The success of recreation services depends more on the quality of leadership than on any other single factor."

In spite of such resounding agreement the lack of a qualified fitness leader is most often the cause of an unsuccessful fitness program. Too often firms immediately consider what kind of equipment they need rather than the leaders who will direct the program. Then well meaning managers guided by the advice of product salesmen with little or no training in physical education, develop and conduct a fitness program. As a result the fitness program is inadequate. Usually only the employees who are already involved in regular exercise even use the equipment. Others make the same mistakes on the company equipment that have caused them to be unfit in the first place. In the end the company joins the list of the many companies that have fancy exercise facilities and only a few users.

Depending on the specific program, a fitness leader might be a full-time, part-time, or volunteer worker. A leader might also be contracted from an outside professional agency. A full-time fitness leader or director should be responsible for organizing and implementing the entire fitness program. Contracted professionals or part-time directors might be used to start the program and for initial fitness testing. Part-time leaders and or volunteer exercise leaders can be used to lead group sessions or to monitor peak use activities after a program has started. In all cases the individual leaders must possess the qualities and characteristics of a good fitness leader.

If a major employee fitness program is being developed as an ongoing enterprise, the hiring of a full-time fitness director would be an effective beginning. A fitness director can be instrumental in conducting the specific needs analysis and in organizing and scheduling the proper solutions. He or she will conduct the fitness testing and retesting and will act as liaison with medical staff for exercise and special program prescriptions. The fitness director should develop an ongoing system of education for the employees, provide personal counseling in all of the many health and fitness related areas, and maintain orderly records on the status of all participants and the program in general. Most importantly the director should coordinate and implement continuous motivational techniques and campaigns.

Although these tasks could be accomplished by hiring someone on a consulting basis, if someone is found who meets the qualifications of a good fitness director, every attempt should be made to bring such a person into the organization permanently.

Qualifications

A fitness leader should be a person who is both inspired and inspiring. He or she should be a product of the product. Not only should the individual's appearance be exemplary of good health and fitness but the philosophy of life should be equally representative. The individual should be intellectually and emotionally involved in those matters most vital in the human condition. The leader should be uniquely gifted in his or her ability to get all sorts of personalities to respond positively to an enthusiastic lead. The person should be receptive, without being "wishy-washy," to new ideas, with a deep respect for and understanding of all living creatures.

Furthermore the individual should represent an attempt to live life to his or her full mental, physical, and creative potential. Life should mean more to the fitness leader than just exercise and fitness. The director should be well rounded with a good sense of humor.

If the above qualifications are not challenging enough, the director should also be knowledgeable about exercise, nutrition, and lifestyle considerations conducive to good health. He should at least be a certified fitness specialist from the American College of Sports Medicine, the National Y.M.C.A. Cardiovascular fitness program, or another respected program. Preferably he or she will also be educated in exercise physiology, physical education administration, and teaching business management. The person should also be qualified in cardiopulmonary resusditation. Although this educational background is significant John Gardner's statement in *No Easy Victories* is most applicable: "Experts are a dime a dozen, what we need is leadership!"

Where to Look

Finding such a fitness leader in itself can be a challenging task. The first place to look is among the organization's own staff. Although it is unlikely that someone in the organization will meet most of the qualifications of a fitness leader, a person with the right personality traits, leadership abilities, and who looks and lives a healthy lifestyle might be considered for training if a mutual interest exists between the employee and the company. If such a person exists within the company, his or her rapport with the employees may already be demonstrated and the knowledge of personnel and the workings of the organization would be an asset.

It is more likely that an organization will have to look to the outside for a fitness director. Before the solicitation process begins, management should have a planned methodology for interviewing and selecting individuals. Dr. Martin Collis, in his *Canadian Manual on Employee Fitness*, appropriately recommends that a committee be organized to provide balanced input into the difficult task of selection. The committee should include:

- A medical representative from occupational health (or from the community if none are employed).
- Management representative
- Union or employee representative
- Recreation representative if one exists
- Outside expert in the area of physical fitness or employee fitness

The committee itself should have a thorough understanding of the various program needs and the qualifications of a fitness director. Of primary concern should be the individual's versatility and not evidence of expertise in physiology. If possible it would be helpful if the committee could observe an applicant actually lead an exercise class. In viewing such a session the committee will have an opportunity to view how well the applicant can handle various types of people, how inspiring he or she is, and how well he or she understands various exercise techniques and priorities.

Once a methodology for choosing a fitness director is established there are various sources that should be tapped. A job advertisement should be placed in local newspapers. There are many qualified individuals in various walks of life who would love a position with a company as a fitness director. Many of these individuals will be leading fitness classes in health spas, running clubs, schools, or Y.M.C.A.'s at relatively low salaries because of their sincere interest in fitness. A higher paying opportunity to put a number of people in shape and keep them there would be, for them, a chance of a lifetime.

Another source would be the American Association of Fitness Directors in Business and Industry (address is in the Appendix) for a list of qualified individuals who might be available. The Association has an employment service that accepts resumes from prospective fitness directors. They will also publish your announcement in their newsletter.

Another source of applicants are the colleges and universities that offer programs in physical education. In searching this avenue it is important that the type of program be evaluated, as many school physical education programs are inadequate preparation for physical fitness directing. Such programs teach little about fitness, lifestyle, and nutrition, and concentrate mainly on games and sports.

A more appropriate graduate might be from a graduate program in exercise physiology. These individuals would have the proper knowledge of exercise, fitness testing principles, and procedures. It would then only be necessary to find the individual with the right personality and leadership characteristics.

At present there are only a few colleges and universities that offer courses in physical fitness leadership. One program exists at Oral Roberts University. Another in Toronto, at the George Brown College of Applied Arts and Technology, offers a two-year Fitness Instructor Diploma. Similarly there are only a few schools that offer degree programs in nutrition and alternative health care. North American College in San Rafael, California, offers certification in fitness, stress management, and nutrition as well as a Masters' Degree in Holistic Health Science. In the near future there should be more schools providing such specialized curriculum.

8

MANAGING TO MOTIVATE

Motivating people to change living habits that have taken years to form is not an easy task. It is especially difficult because the motivational objectives that surround the quest for health and fitness have been filled with confusion and negative responses. The failure to practice healthy living habits is more a result of a "demotivating campaign" than the result of ignorance, laziness, or apathy.

The misguiding factors have been described in detail elsewhere in this book, but deserve mention here because they must be understood before motivational efforts are made. These factors include cultural and educational emphasis on sports instead of lifelong exercise, military service physical fitness training, and cultural discouragement of exercise for women.

Fitness leaders will also have to appreciate the existence of influences that promote a dependence on the medical system for health care. Medication for high blood pressure, drug prescriptions for sleeplessness, and surgery for heart disease are but a few revered recommendations that are subversive of health.

Commercial and institutional influences must also be considered while attempting to motivate people to change their lifestyle. Values have been confused by an emphasis on wealth and convenience. For every attempt to motivate people to reduce their sugar intake, the media will make a dozen attempts to motivate people to consume sugar. In many instances, motivating people to participate in a fitness program depends on the more difficult task of motivating people to change their values and institutions.

Variety of Motives

Motivating people to start and stay with a fitness program is thus a challenging proposition. Not only must the attempt contend with powerful cultural and social influences, but individual personality, psychological characteristics, age, and sex, are material as well.

For example, there is often a difference between motivating executives and hourly wage earners. Executives are more willing to participate in a fitness program but have problems adjusting priorities to allot time. One company offered an employee fitness program, but only twenty percent of the hourly wage earners participated as compared to sixty percent of the executives.

This illustration does not indicate that people or motives can necessarily be categorized. Not only will different people respond to different approaches, but motives for a single person may vary from time to time. As new moralities, new awareness, new interests, and new needs arise, new motivations will be applicable as well.

The aim should thus be to develop a motivational campaign that provides the greatest variety of motives for the largest number of people. If specific needs indicate specific motives for significant populations, then appropriate efforts should be made. There is, however, seldom enough time, energy, or resources to address all the needs of all individuals.

The variety of motivational alternatives is as wide as the variety of behavioral influences. Some companies award colored T-shirts that indicate accumulated hours of exercise. One company displays a map with strings attached from point to point to indicate distance and routes run or walked by various individuals. Others have computer terminals for personal progress information. One company advertised a reported improvement in sexual activities to motivate employees.

Monthly slogans and posters are also used effectively to stimulate a variety of responses. Examples include, "Warning—continued use of elevators may be hazardous to your health," "Ride now—pay later," "You can't sit and be fit," "Never trust a thought you arrive at sitting down," and others.

The number of motivational techniques is limited only by imagination. There are, however, ten concepts that are fundamental to most kinds of fitness motivation. As these concepts are considered, it should be noted that for each positive influence evoked by applying a motivational technique that embraces the concept, a negative response is also possible. The emotional aspects of fitness and employment policies can be precarious. For this reason most techniques should be implemented only after management has displayed a responsive, sincere concern for the health and welfare of employees and after demonstrating a commitment and belief in the benefits of fitness. The motivational concepts relate to the following ten areas.

- The prevention of illness and death and/or the acquisition of optimal health.
- Rewards and recognition
- Peer pressure, social participation and comaraderie
- Penalties and retribution
- Competition
- Testing
- Leadership and Supervision
- Company time for program
- Enjoyment
- The self concept

For the Health of It

According to Dr. Kenneth Cooper, the two best incentives to exercise are (1) if a friend the same age has had a heart attack and (2) if a person himself has a chest pain and is unsure as to what caused it. A third might be if someone has had a heart attack, has survived without serious impairment, and sincerely believes that an exercise program would diminish the chances of having another one.

Unfortunately such cases represent the few occasions when people exercise to prevent illness or death. As with most preventive measures, efforts are usually commensurate with the immediacy of the problem that is to be prevented.

The truth is that most people do not enter into a fitness program just "for the health of it." There are many reasons for this. It is human nature to take the easiest path with only the short term in mind. It is easier not to exercise and diet in the short term. In spite of evidence to the contrary, if there is no immediate penalty for not exercising, or smoking, or not eating properly, there is no perceived need to exercise.

Immediate gratification resulting from improved fitness can be realized only in subtle degrees. The feeling of relaxation after exercising, the ability to sleep better, and revitalization are realized only after a person begins exercising. To stimulate this realization before the fact requires consistent and meaningful education.

This is all not to say that health is not important to people. It is that people take their bodies for granted. No financial transaction was required to purchase the body and monthly payments do not reflect an investment in health. There is no thought of maintenance for resale. Health care costs are indirect until it is too late. Until the social system taxes people for having symptoms of poor fitness, an educational campaign will have to teach people not to take their health for granted. Such a campaign existed in the 1950s with regard to dental health.

One way that management can implement the prevention motive is to begin to identify conditions that significantly increase health risks. Each month a new factor can be emphasized with posters, lectures, and newsletters. For example, relationships should be drawn between back pain and weak muscles, between diet and diabetes, between cancer and environmental carcinogens, or between symptoms and diseases of inactivity.

Questionnaires can be used to stimulate an awareness of health risks. Some people really have not thought about the number of drugs they consume, or the hours that they are inactive. Questionnaires or health hazard appraisals like the one presented in Chapter Nine can be used.

Within a campaign to motivate people to enter programs to prevent illness or premature death should be reference to the benefits of optimal health, i.e., that degree of health that goes beyond mere absence of disease. Promotion of this idea might publicize pictures of the special vitality, opportunities, and tranquility that can come from such health. Reference to older Americans who are exceptionally active (see Chapter 14) are useful for this end.

If a business is successful enough to be considering employee fitness programs in the first place, it probably has the tools and talent for product or service promotion. If a company can make people believe that smoking cigarettes will simulate the rugged outdoor existence and that drinking cola will bring happiness, then a company can also make people believe that regular physical activity and lifestyle modification can be very worthwhile.

Although there will be people who are already receptive to motivation that stresses both the quality of and the quantity of years of life, it will take a while before such considerations are motivational to most people. In the meantime it should be remembered that personal health is a sensitive subject and people dislike insinuations that they may be unhealthy. Promotions should be educational, not directional.

Rewards and Recognition

Another way to motivate employees to participate in fitness programs is with positive incentives. Trophies, awards, T-shirts, and such often have the same appeal for adults as the gold star has had for children. The President's Council on Physical Fitness and Sports has a sports award program that offers participants patches for accomplishing a certain amount of activity in a variety of sports. Forms for this and log books for the various sports can be obtained for free by writing to the Council in Washington, D.C.

Awards can be given by the company for hours logged or for percentage of improvement in fitness measurements. One company sends key executives to an expensive health spa for two weeks on the condition that they regularly attend the company program on their return. The same company provides further positive incentives by running a well organized program that offers a variety of indoor-outdoor facilities.

The idea of paying employees for improvements in fitness has merit, considering the potential economic return. Dr. Godfrey M. Hockbaum, Professor of Health Education and Behavioral Science in the School of Public Health at the University of North Carolina, agrees. He believes that employers should be persuaded to raise salaries of employees who observe preventative rules for good health.

Several firms have already implemented this idea. Speedball Corporation, an electronics manufacturer, pays their employees seven dollars a week for not smoking on the job. Lowes, Inc. of Cassopolis, Michigan, pays one and one half percent of the employee's annual salary if an executive can lose one pound per week until his or her ideal weight is attained.

Although the financial incentives for fitness in business and industry can and should be used in some cases to motivate people, management must recognize the possible negative repercussions of such a policy. There have been cases where pay incentives were challenged by employee groups as being unfair. Although there is not justification for this, it must be remembered that the goal of management is to spark interest, not resentment. Also, it is possible that the financial incentive might obscure the real value of fitness and in the long run may not be effective.

The Social Motives

The social motives for entering a fitness program include a desire for social participation and peer pressure. Fitness programs offer an opportunity to become better acquainted with fellow employees. They offer a rare and important chance for interaction between management and regular employees. It is also easier to commit oneself to an exercise session if it is done with friends and fellow employees. On the other side of the coin, not participating with fellow employees may lead to an uncomfortable co-existence with participating employees.

The opportunity to become socially involved with others can be an important incentive. A government survey in Britain found that "a chance to mix with people" was a major reason why women chose to participate in fitness programs. Organizers can emphasize this motive in numerous ways. Creative posters describing the social benefits can be made. For example, "Employees that play together will work together better." Social activities can follow occasional exercise sessions, and recreational activities can be used as occasional alternatives as long as they incorporate the fitness principles and discourage aggressive competition.

The employees involved in one company fitness program formed a social committee to help maintain a high level of participation. If someone drops out of the program, members of the committee informally and formally try to encourage the person to return with references to the social comrade philosophy. "We miss you," "You were doing so well, you were helping me," "It's not the same without you," etc., are approaches that exemplify such tactics.

Negative peer pressure can be as successful as the positive peer pressure. *Forbes* magazine has a motivation policy whereby employees participating in their fitness program gently admonish their colleagues who do not attend regularly. Management can stimulate negative peer pressure by suggesting that program benefits may be curtailed if there is not an increase in participants. It can also be suggested that salary increases may be dependent on reductions in health insurance premiums, which in turn may be reduced if a majority of employees become fit. Such tactics may cause employee leaders to emerge and peer pressure may encourage everyone to participate.

Another way to implement the peer pressure motive is to aim promotional efforts at people who most often associate with the target employee. For example, instead of trying to encourage an employee to exercise directly, an associate can be encouraged to motivate him or her. This idea is illustrated by the slogan, "Have you ever thought how nice it would be to work with a healthy associate?" or, "Is your partner a hazard to your health?" or, "Is someone else's smoke ruining your health?"

Such indirect efforts can also be aimed at associations outside the workplace. Spouses can be encouraged to motivate their mates via letters and invitations to participate in program functions. Other family members and friends can be involved as well. At Xerox the program facility is available to all the members of an employee's family. For single employees, rules allow their friends to use the facility.

The possible negative aspects of social motivation should also be understood. Non-participating employees, if threatened by the specific technique employed, may ban together to apply peer pressure *not* to participate in fitness programs. A person may be singled out as a "traitor" or "fitness freak." A demonstrated commitment to fitness by management personnel can usually keep this type of peer pressure to a minimum.

Jealousy can also be evoked within the social setting if peer pressure tactics are inappropriate. As people improve fitness levels and their appearance and attitudes improve, others may become envious and resentful. People may also be jealous of the fact that someone else has managed to attain the motivation to stay with a program where they have failed. It is an unfortunate fact of human nature that people often become resentful of those who are happy and successful, but such attitudes can be kept to a minimum with the right motivational approaches and support.

Spouses can also be a barrier. If only one spouse is motivated to participate, the other may feel antagonistic toward the changes and lack of personal involvement. More time may be spent away from home by the participant in new activities. Dinners that are prepared with love, but with unhealthy foods, may be rejected by the newly educated participant. If spouses are not motivated by management to participate in a healthy lifestyle with their mates, withdrawal from a fitness program may seem more appropriate than a divorce.

Another possible negative aspect of social motivation has to do with the group participation programs that are for both male and female employees. Men or women who are not in good shape are often self-conscious about their appearance before members of the opposite sex, especially during exercise sessions. Before a co-educational program is implemented, management should verify that the majority of employees are in favor of such a program.

Negative Based Incentives

Penalties for "incorrect behavior" have long been considered powerful motivators. Demotions, salary deductions, penalty fees, and browbeating for not being fit, however, will have little success in instigating employee fitness programs. Although such things might be put into a condition of employment contract when someone is first hired, a barrage of grievances and civil suits would result if such a tactic were used by management. Furthermore, even those employees interested in fitness would resent such control by management. Although such tactics might be justified in certain professions, they should be avoided in most business and industry situations.

There are some other negative based incentives that might be motivational to a large number of people without significant negative repercussions. "Fear tactics" that emphasize the potential harm caused by not participating could be used if benefit tactics seem to be missing impact. For example, anti-smoking posters can be obtained from the American Cancer Society that graphically depict the horror of mouth cancer. Kimberly Clark has a program physician who lays the hard facts on the line to employees during their health examinations. Dr. Robert A. Dedmon, staff vice-president of Medical Affairs for Kimberly Clark, says that telling a forty year old mailroom clerk he has the body of a sixty-three year old makes the person sit up and take notice.

Another negative based policy is the establishment of tough rules about attendance in the fitness program. A failure to participate a minimum number of hours per week can result in immediate suspension from the program. Such strict rules can be imposed in conjunction with an intentional pilot program that limits the number of employees in such a way that there will always be a waiting list, at least in the first year. Such a restriction can have the effect of creating an increased demand for the program only because access is more difficult.

A similar incentive that can both motivate people to exercise and help pay for the program is to charge a fee for fitness program privileges. Marketing research has demonstrated that chances of the success of a product or service sometimes increase with an increase in the price of the item. The same item that failed to sell well at five dollars might sell exceptionally well if sold for ten. This same psychology can be applied to increasing the value attached to the fitness program.

Before scare tactics or financial costs are used as a motivational tool, a careful analysis of employee attitudes should determine if it is the best course. Monthly attendance rates can be compared using both techniques as well as using a combination of the two to see which approach or combination seems effective. A nominal charge very often will not discourage those who resent paying for the service and may be enough to motivate someone who would not be interested if the program were free.

Competition

The desire to compete is often the only reason a person exercises.

Being "in training" may be the only reason a person refrains from excessive alcohol or cigarette smoking. Competitiveness may be inherent in human nature, and as such can have a significant motivational impact when used appropriately. The spirit of competition, for example, is frequently used in motivating salespeople to increase their sales.

Competitive motivations are especially applicable to the executive personality. Rival company competition oriented toward fitness is already gaining widespread popularity. A new annual event called the Tyler Cup sponsors running relays between businesses. Last year the Dallas based event attracted one hundred thirty businesses from eleven different states. Forty corporation teams entered the Chicago Distance classic the same year. In New York seventy-two companies competed in races called the "Summer Corporate Challenges" sponsored by Manufacturers Hanover.

Destined to be the largest fitness promotion competitions between corporations are the Corporate Cup Relays. The Corporate Cup Relays are a series of seven regional meets that culminate with a national championship event. They are sponsored by *Runner's World* magazine and are conducted by the Corporate Cup Association, an organization of companies of all sizes committed to "promoting the fitness and health of employees by sponsoring competitive athletic events among member companies." The intent of the races is to "demonstrate how companies can provide team sport competition for employees who have completed their formal schooling and presently have no framework within which to continue such competition."

The traditional popularity of competition may prompt a fitness director to implement this form of motivation without careful consideration of its possible negative aspects. Care should be taken that this does not happen. The competitive motive can be as responsible for people not exercising as it is for people exercising. The difference will depend on the attitudes and atmosphere that surround the competition.

The emphasis on competition has been a negative influence on fitness for several reasons. First of all, the stressing of maximum performance creates an intensity of participation that cannot be maintained for many years. Secondly, the emphasis on competition is too often on winning, not on the benefits of health and the perfection of abilities. And third, as the joy of winning has been exclaimed, so has the disappointment of losing. For many the stigma of "losing" a competition is not worth the gamble.

One solution to overcoming the negative aspects of competition is to create scoreless competitive type events. Volleyball games can be played between teams with the objective of seeing how many times the ball can legally be exchanged over the net. Racquetball competition can be played to see how many times the ball can be hit without reservation before someone misses it. Such games can give the opportunity for competitive action without the win-lose syndrome.

Another way to overcome the negative aspects is by providing handicaps based on athletic experience, fitness levels, sex, or time trials. When handicaps are given and the goal of fitness is the obvious objective, people who would otherwise be unwilling to compete often become involved.

The third solution, and perhaps the best, is to promote a proper attitude about competition. People can be re-educated to understand that there is a difference between competing to win and competing to measure one's ability and training level. Using scoring and competing against others is a natural way to push oneself to see how close one is to a potential. Some sports competition can help people know one another, both as opponents and as teammates. The sport of ride and tie is a good example of how competition can create a bond between opposing teams. Boxers hugging each other after ten rounds of aggressive fighting are another illustration of how competition can be rewarding if doing one's best remains more important than winning. With this type of understanding in mind, losing is only a disappointment when one has participated at a level below current capability. If one's capability was reached, losing is then only a measurement for future training objectives.

Before competitive motives are implemented in a company, the slogan, "It's not whether you win or lose, it's how you play the game" should be a sincere belief by all participants and prospective participants.

Testing

One of the ten motivational concepts basic to employee fitness participation has to do with the use of fitness testing. Testing is a method of motivation that has long been used in schools. Although Chapter 9 will deal with this subject thoroughly, it should be mentioned here that testing is an educational tool as well as a motivational tool. If the emphasis is on prescribed standards instead of a measurable basis for determining progress, then the use of testing can become a negative motivator.

Testing is also important in as much as it provides goals for people. The need for goals is an important human need that is ignored often in modern society. There are many goals that can be achieved by improving fitness. The goals need not be directly related to the fitness measurements. They might have to do with completing a marathon or a three mile run. They might be hiking through the Grand Canyon or giving someone a good game of tennis. Whatever goals and objectives are chosen, they should be attainable. The objective of goal-oriented motivation should stimulate thought about the attainment of such goals.

Direction

Sometimes the best promotion a product or service can get is no more than a reputation for excellence. If the employee fitness program possesses that excellence, little more may be required to keep members involved. As participants spread the word it will not be long before others will want to join.

According to several surveys, proper direction and supervision of a fitness program and its facilities were a major factor in assuring program adherence. A fitness program is like any other educational program. If the educators are inadequate, people will drop out. If they are good, people will learn and grow. For this reason all members of the fitness program management staff should be continually trained by the fitness director in program development and maintenance skills. Their approach to fitness supervision should remain enthusiastic, varied, and knowledgeable.

Everyone involved with supervising actual exercise sessions should encourage an enjoyable, informal atmosphere. Fitness instructors should maintain a sense of humor while dealing with participants. During group exercise there should be a continual flow of activity, but every effort should be made to give individual attention to various participants. This is especially important during the first six weeks of participation in a program when the attrition rate is usually the highest.

Consistency is another important variable in assuring quality supervision. Fitness leaders should not be expected to know everything about nutrition, physiology, and lifestyle. When they do not know an answer, however, it is important that they do not guess or give a personal opinion without qualifying it as such. If this is allowed, various answers to questions will confuse participants and they may lose faith in the program.

The program should also be consistent with corporate management policies and working conditions. Cafeteria menus should provide a variety of choices including foods that comply with the nutritional recommendations of Chapter 2. Cigarette and candy machines should be removed from the premises. Special sections should be set aside for smokers and no smoking should be allowed in working areas. Conferences and meetings should enforce no smoking rules and should have exercise breaks when appropriate. The use of stairs in place of elevators should be encouraged and practiced. Other inconsistencies with health maintenance should be avoided as part of the supervisory responsibilities.

A quality program is also influenced by a reinforcement of fitness principles by company management. There should be continual cooperation between company management and the fitness program management. This should include everything from maintaining the attractiveness of the facilities to facilitating payroll deductions for program membership.

Company management should also be encouraged to participate visibly in the program. Such participation reinforces the program significantly. The practicing of that which is preached is an imperative if the program is to remain credible. If the company leaders do not display a sincere commitment to the program, subordinates will surely hesitate at program involvement.

Company Time

Employees participating in Exxon's New York fitness program were surveyed to determine what was the most important factor in program adherence. The fact that the program allowed participation during working hours was reported as the most important factor in the prevention of dropout. Although most company fitness programs are conducted around working hours, the investment return of such a policy is often minimal compared to what it could be otherwise.

Using the other motivational concepts can, of course, bring a significant number of employees into the program. The difficulty, however, of motivating people to leave for work an hour early, stay an hour longer, or omit their lunch break to exercise is much greater than motivating people to take an hour out of their work routine. The mere fact that employees can participate on company time and are getting paid for participating is extremely motivating.

Management should be convinced that if scheduling can accommodate it, the hour's time away from work duties will not necessarily decrease productivity. In fact, in many occupations the work slowdown from fatigue can be eliminated by a fitness program and work productivity can increase. In assembly line situations where an employee may not be able to leave his or her post for as much as an hour, a ten minute exercise break in the morning and in the afternoon can revitalize and may prevent accidents and mistakes. Since such breaks will not be intense enough to make significant aerobic improvements, a regular program should also be offered around working hours.

Giving an employee credit for being able to organize and complete his or her working duties is in itself an inspiration to participate in the company encouraged program. Such an acknowledgement will improve employee morale; when morale improves participation in a fitness program is more likely. Many European companies provide on-sight distractions from the work routine because the energy gained from such distractions has been found to go back into the job. One company in Germany shows Laurel and Hardy movies during the day.

If time is given to employees during the working hours for exercise, care should be taken that the opportunity is not abused by some individuals so as to jeopardize the opportunity for all. A maximum number of hours per week should be set at three. (This should also be a recommended minimum of total hours spent exercising.) Scheduling and provisions should be made so utilization is spread out throughout the day and business areas are not left unattended.

Once the scheduling is implemented, administrative support for the idea should be widely publicized. In many cases employees might feel guilty exercising during work hours even though it has been officially approved. This is especially true when facilities exist outside the building. The outdoors is a great motivator for exercise, but employees must overcome the guilt of leaving the building during working hours. The goal of motivational efforts should be to make employees feel responsible and proud for participating, not guilty or apprehensive.

If it is impossible to provide on-duty time for exercise, there should at least be opportunities for employees to occasionally get together and discuss exercise information and experiences. There should also be occasional seminars or lectures during company time. At the very least, there should be five or ten minute exercise breaks. And, most importantly, there should be an effective motivational campaign to get employees to participate before or after work or during their lunch break.

Enjoyability

The fact that regular exercise cannot always be an enjoyable activity has been discussed previously. The required intensity and regularity prohibits most people from choosing a completely enjoyable alternative for each session. Although boredom and dislike must be kept to a minimum, modern lifestyles dictate that less preferable alternatives be used periodically. An artificial society requires artificial physical activity if natural health and natural activities are to remain possibilities.

Next to the "self concept," however, enjoyability is the most influential motivational concept. Without the "revolution of play" referred to by Dr. George Sheehan, the fitness revolution becomes meaningless. Before fitness can become a goal, fitness must have a goal and enjoyment of life may be the ultimate goal. Thus, if enjoyability can be attached to a fitness program, a maximum rate of participation and adherence can be expected.

A 1973 Nielsen survey rated activities that promoted physical fitness as to their degree of enjoyability. Swimming was rated as number one and bicycling number two. Unfortunately, neither of these activities are usually feasible in an employee fitness program, especially on a year-round basis. Although they should be implemented where possible, surveys should determine the preference of those alternatives that are feasible within the company environment.

The pursuit of enjoyable fitness activities usually leads to the development of recreational activities. Since it has been stressed that most recreational activities do not properly promote fitness, care should be taken that recreational activities be modified so that they incorporate the basic principles of fitness achievement. Games can be invented so that continuous, safe, and fun cardiovascular exercises can be achieved.

There are many motivational techniques that can make fitness fun. The moans and groans and jokes are a typical part of most team sport calisthenics sessions. Fun posters, enjoyable music, colorful surroundings, sociable camaraderie, and interesting exercises can all contribute to the enjoyment of a fitness program.

Another way to put fun in a program is to provide guest speakers and films that are stimulating and related to fitness. Employees themselves can be used as speakers to discuss their hobbies or changes in life their fitness has instigated.

Fitness expeditions can also be scheduled for weekends that fall during the regular exercise sessions. A skiing trip, a hiking trip, a group run, and many other enjoyable activities can be scheduled and used as a motivating resource.

If swimming pools, sports activities that promote fitness, and other intrinsically enjoyable activities can be used to implement an employee fitness program, so much the better. The primary goal is to make the fitness program, whatever its design, an enjoyable experience.

The Self Concept

Although the preceding concepts provide a basis for understanding and applying motivational strategies, motivation cannot be considered a straightforward process. As a science, behavior modification is still in its infancy. Psychology itself remains an ongoing study of human needs, consciousness, growth, achievement, and significance. An attempt to motivate is an attempt to understand human nature and its complexities. More than that, it is an attempt to control one or more of these complexities. Perhaps this is one reason so little is known about motivation.

Motivation is, of course, possible. People are motivated to do something every day. Furthermore, motivation is not the exclusive domain of psychologists. Motivational techniques are successfully implemented by advertisers, salesmen, school teachers, athletic coaches, parents, and children. The objectives of these people, however, are usually simplistic compared to those of a fitness director.

In spite of the somewhat more challenging goal of fitness motivation, all of the above motivational situations play upon one singular desire. That desire is to make the "self concept" real, i.e., to live in a manner that is appropriate to or symbolic of one's preferred role. A person buys an expensive car because it is appropriate to his or her preferred image. A father finally stops his busy schedule or interrupts his nap to play with his little girl because his role demands it. A man may begin exercising so that he might look well on the beach and participate in a role he has long desired.

How motivated a person is to do something depends on how much of a chance he or she believes there is to realize a portion of the preferred role. The objective of fitness motivation should thus be to convince people that their preferred roles can be achieved with exercise and healthy lifestyle changes. Since many basic human needs including physiological needs, safety, esteem, and self improvement, can often be satisfied by improving fitness, there is great potential for successful fitness motivation. For example, a primary reason for exercising given by women who participate in fitness programs is to improve their figure.

Still, most people do not practice healthy behavior. The relationship between fitness and the basic human needs is frustrating and ironical because it is not rational. What of the many women with poor figures who do not exercise? What of the people who most need physiological assistance, self-esteem, and self-improvement? Why is it so difficult for a person to understand that many preferred roles can be obtained through a change in lifestyle?

The answer given to these questions throughout this text is that people have not been properly educated. The "self concept," however, addresses a more profound personal solution. If a person has never achieved a preferred role, he or she will have developed many defenses to avoid the disappointment of that failure. In many cases education cannot erase those defenses. Even if it could, a person is apprehensive that a serious commitment toward the attainment of that role could end in failure. Such a commitment would require the dissolution of defenses that had been established, and a return to reality after such a failure could be a psychological trauma.

The failure to make a long-term and logical commitment by such individuals is partly responsible for the success of product advertisements that claim superficial, short-term, and illogical commitments will give a person an opportunity to live a preferred role. All that is necessary to become a rugged individualist, an adventurer, a loving family person, the life of a party, or a glamorous sex symbol is the purchase of a particular brand of beer, a pack of cigarettes, a bouquet of flowers, a breath mint, or a girdle. The success of instant fat loss schemes and products is also an example of a person striking out after a desired role without risking emotional stakes and failures.

The personal solution to this predicament is in demonstrating that a person is capable of attaining his or her preferred role without failure. A fitness leader must instill faith within an individual that he or she cannot fail. A person may be confined to a wheelchair, with the potentiality to walk again and a list of emotional safeguards that have allowed him to tolerate the impairment. Such a person may be unwilling to even attempt rehabilitation because of a lack of faith and a resultant fear of failure. Once some degree of faith is stimulated, the person may learn to walk.

The best way to instill this faith is through the process of "minor successes." A fitness director must guide a person into some activity where success in the short term is guaranteed and where a minimum commitment is necessary. Once success is attained in that activity, progressively more difficult activities are encouraged until self-confidence and faith in one's ability to be successful is established. The process of minor success as it relates to the attainment of health, self-esteem, and well-being will be discussed further in Part Three.

9

TOOLS FOR TESTING

This chapter will present a complete protocol for individual fitness evaluations. Its intent is to provide a comprehensive methodology useful to everyone involved with supervising a fitness program.

The appropriateness of providing laymen with a methodology for conducting fitness testing is in keeping with the desire to take responsibility for health care away from the professional and give it to the individual. Although it is preferable for a company to have a fitness specialist initially conduct fitness testing for insurance purposes and the advantages of professional experience, participants can eventually learn to test themselves. In some cases it may not be feasible for a company to hire a professional and a leader will emerge from management or the ranks who will need the information contained herein.

There are several advantages to self-administered fitness evaluations. Individuals can test themselves as often as they choose, at times most appropriate to their fitness progression. Time and scheduling difficulties can be avoided if a fitness director does not have to do all the testing, although he can help supervise self-testing procedures. A third advantage is that employees who test themselves might not experience the apprehension, embarrassment, and guilt associated with being tested by someone else.

It should be noted that this third consideration also has a negative side. In some cases the motivating aspect of fitness testing relates not only to identifying improvements in fitness but also to the obligation to be tested and the opportunity to impress the fitness director performing the tests. The Weight Watcher program illustrates this point. They require that their members report and be weighed weekly; this requirement is largely responsible for the success of their program. Obviously the members could weigh themselves at home and save their money, but the fact that someone else is doing it, and the obligation to participate, are influential in causing an adherence to the weight loss program.

In any case the motivational aspect of fitness testing is significant if properly administered. Dr. Manuel Cooper found that fitness testing was the best motivator for participants in the Boeing Company fitness program. Twenty percent of their people quit smoking just from seeing how bad their condition was compared to standards for their age.

If fitness evaluations are to be safe and motivational it is essential that the technician be thoroughly competent. Since the protocols described in this chapter do not require sophisticated equipment, electronic knowledge, or medical interpretation, years of training are not necessary. There is, however, a need for measurement proficiency to assure accuracy and consistency, a knowledge of the purpose of the specific tests, an awareness of the hazards of the test, and an ability to prevent, recognize, and treat overuse, exhaustion, or coronary repercussions.

The person administering the fitness tests should also help to serve the four functions of the tests. These functions include motivation, education, prescription, and diagnostic capabilities.

The tester should be pleasant and display a sense of humor without expressing ridicule. The tester should also be able to read the participant's potential reaction to norm comparisons. Some people are demoralized if their own fitness measurement is far below the "good" or "average" ratings. Others are encouraged to improve such scores. The best way to handle the combined curiosity to know where one stands, and the discouragement of finding out, is to show a person their relative fitness score but emphasize that the ratings and norms are highly subjective and that the only thing that is important is an improvement on one's score, whatever it is.

The educational aspect of testing may be the most important responsibility of a tester. The fitness evaluations on most field tests are not highly accurate physiological measurements. For example, reliable improvements can be monitored using percentage of fat measurements, yet they are usually several percentages away from being physiologically exact. Still, the conceptual understanding of fat loss and its relationship to body mass is gained from the taking of a percentage of fat measurement. The more informative, instructional, and receptive to questions a tester is, the greater will be the educational experience.

The fitness test should also provide a basis for exercise prescription. The measurements may indicate that more work is needed on improving flexibility than on improving strength, for example. Cardiovascular exercise alternatives and intensities can also be recommended depending on aerobic fitness scores. If an individual has a very low score, it is more important for that person to proceed with cardiovascular exercises gradually and at the lower percentage of maximum heart rate. (See "Training Heart Rate" in the Appendix).

The most convenient protocol for exercise prescription based on the fitness tests included in this chapter is for the fitness director to attach the scores to four general classifications. A form (next page) will be sufficient for most programs not using initial medical evaluations and screening.

The diagnostic value of the fitness tests in this chapter are primarily limited to spirometry, blood pressure, and the lifestyle evaluation. These tests may reveal respiratory illness, hypertension, and coronary risk factors. The diagnostic value of fitness evaluation is more properly reserved for physicians and more elaborate equipment.

Another reason that fitness testing should be highly efficient has to do with the contribution of evidence to the national effort. In terms of proving that physical fitness has a money payoff to business and industry, and in terms of showing that employee fitness programs can significantly improve the health and longevity of people, properly organized protocols, record keeping, and coordination between testing and program implementation are essential.

Although various protocols have been developed by universities, Y.M.C.A.s, and other organizations, as well as the one included in this book, whatever protocol is chosen must remain consistent from one evaluation to the next. The protocol should also include all of the basic measurements including aerobic capacity (oxygen uptake), flexibility, muscle strength and endurance, body composition and measurements, and blood pressure.

Canada has gone one step further in the attempt to make a contribution to their national health. Their Health and Welfare Department has devised a simple testing protocol with the recommendation that it be considered the standard protocol for all non-clinical fitness tests. It includes a step test, anthropometric measurements, flexibility, muscular strength and endurance, and pulmonary function.

Another way to augment the growth of fitness data that will support the national and international movement is to supplement

Personal
Fitness Testing Clinic

NAME _____ SEX _____ DATE _____

BIRTHDATE _____ AGE____ WEIGHT ____ HEIGHT ___

Examiner	Measure	Score	Limit
_____	Resting Heart Rate	_____ Beats/Min.	Over 100
_____	Resting Systolic Blood Pressure	_____ MM HG	Over 150 Over 100
_____	Resting Diastolic Blood Pressure	_____ MM HG	Over 100
_____	Vital Capacity (VC)	_____ Liters	
_____	Forced Expiratory Volume (FEV1)	_____ Liters	
_____	FEV1, % of VC (% VC Total)	_____ %	Below 80%
_____	Trunk Flexion	_____	
_____	Grip Strength	_____	
_____	Body Composition	_____	
_____	Physical Capacity Test	_____	
_____	Maximum O2 Uptake	_____	
_____	Pulse Recovery	_____	

Notes:

the field testing with more elaborate testing. Such tests might include use of a Cybex machine, ECG equipment, blood chemistry analysis for cholesterol, triglycerides, HDL/LDH ratio, and many other bodily functions that might relate to health maintenance. Within the next few years most of the expected contributions of exercise and diet will be measurable with highly accurate technical innovations. Such physiological benefits can be categorized according to the systems of the body as follows:

Musculoskeletal System:

- Active bones and ligaments are strengthened.
- Calcirication of bones is increased.
- Cartilages are thickened.
- Flexibility is improved.
- Muscle strength and volume are increased.
- Capillary density is increased.
- Fat in muscle tissue is reduced.
- Enzymatic changes occur in cells.

Cardiovascular System:

- Heart rate lowered.
- Stroke volume increased.
- Blood volume increased.
- Heart volume increased.
- Capillary density increased.
- Hemoglobin increased.
- Cardiac output increased.

Respiratory System:

- Lung volume changes (only in extreme cases).
- Chest musculature can be increased.
- Patterns of breathing may be altered.
- Ability to extract oxygen is improved.

Central Nervous System:

- Quicker reaction time.
- More efficient mechanical response.
- More rapid response to postural changes.

Once a significant data bank of evidence that is acceptable to the medical and scientific community is established for verifying the above changes, it will be easier to convince business, community, and health leaders of the importance of organizing fitness programs.

Much of this responsibility is in the hands of the fitness testing technician or the fitness director.

The Evaluations

The information contained in this chapter may be all that is necessary to provide a comprehensive battery of evaluations with which to begin and measure the progress of an employee fitness program. The function, procedures, and equipment related to each test will be described. Equipment costs will vary from around two hundred dollars for the least expensive alternatives to around two thousand dollars or less for the most expensive. The protocols described include comparative norms for most of the following measurements:

- lifestyle evaluation
- resting heart rate
- resting blood pressure
- anthropometric measurements
- body composition
- spirometry
- cardiorespiratory endurance (aerobic capacity)
- exercise recovery rate
- flexibility
- muscular strength and endurance

Also included in this chapter is a "Fitness Measurement Worksheet" and a "Personal Fitness Profile." Other forms and charts that may be used to enhance personal exercise and nutrition programs will be included in the Appendix, including a computation form for determining a training heart rate.

Before the Test

Before testing is begun, the facilities should be organized to assure the greatest expedience. Each station should be located in such a way so that crowding does not occur if more than one person is being tested at one time. The sequence of tests should be such that the strength and endurance tests do not precede the cardiovascular test. Blood pressure and resting heart rates should be taken first of all. Clipboards, stopwatches, and pencils should be available for all technicians. Each participant should carry his or her own "fitness measurement worksheet" from station to station.

Before subjects arrive at the testing area, they should be prepared for taking the tests. Participants should be punctual if group scheduling is necessary. They should wear gym clothes and bring a swim-suit and towel if underwater weighing is being done. They should be reminded not to eat food, drink coffee or alcohol, smoke, or exercise within three hours of the evaluation.

Participants should also know beforehand that the test results are strictly confidential. They should appreciate the fact that the evaluations are for educational purposes. Norms should be regarded as mere guidelines for improvement. Participants should also be informed that progress reports to management and for publication will always be in the aggregate. (Figure 1 shows an aggregate results table for 110 participants in the Exxon fitness program). And fi-nally, all participants should sign an "informed consent" form similar to the one in the Appendix.

Test Number 1: Lifestyle Evaluation

Most health experts agree that today's major health problems result from self-imposed lifestyles and environment. In many cases an individual can do little to change environmental factors. Indus-trial pollution, the automobile, radiation, and other environmental problems can only be minimized by the individual. Their hazards are otherwise unavoidable. Other lifestyle risks are under the control of individuals, and here may lie the greatest tragedies. According to the World Health Organization, for example, control of cigarette smoking would do more to improve the health of people than any other single act in preventive medicine.

An awareness of risk factors and their relationship to sickness and premature death can be enough to motivate some people to begin a fitness program. Improvements in answers to questions concerning lifestyle habits can also be motivational as well as indica-tive of fitness program success.

There are many varieties of lifestyle evaluation questionnaires. The Institute of Health Research in San Francisco uses a twenty-four page format and is interpreted by physicians and computers. Dr. Lewis Robbins developed the "Health Hazard Appraisal" which attaches numbers to a variety of risks to determine potential surviv-al over the next ten years with and without personal lifestyle change. Another computer assessed program is called L.I.F.E. (Lifestyle Inventory, Fitness Evaluation.) It appraises one's "biological age" and makes suggestions for improvement.

The questionnaire presented here for lifestyle evaluation does not require professional interpretation. It merely identifies a number of major health risks. The risks included on this questionnaire are based

Name..................................

Date ....

No. Boxes Checked ....

Lifestyle Evaluation

Statement of Confidentiality

This questionairre is for educational and motivational purposes only, as are all of the evaluations. It will remain strictly confidential and will in no way be considered as part of your employment or personal record. It will be used to measure your progress during the fitness program so that your program can be properly adjusted if necessary.

Rating of Questionaire

The following rating will be used to determine your "Personal Fitness Profile" which will graph your fitness level based on most of the tests. It is categorized for your convenience in measuring improvment and for providing a relative understanding of desirability. The score relates to the number of boxes checked below.

Men:	8-10 . . . (Excellent)	6-7 . . . (Good)	
Women:	10-12 . . . (Excellent)	8 - 9 . . . (Good)	
Men:	4-5 . . . . (Average)	0-3 . . . . (Poor)	
Women:	6 - 7 . . . (Average)	0 - 5 . . . (Poor)	

Directions

Put a check in the box following each statement **only** if it is applicable to your own lifestyle. If the statement is not a valid description of your lifestyle or you don't know the answer, leave the box blank and go on to the next question.

Category	Statement	Applicability (check if true)
Smoking	I do not smoke (includes cigarettes, pipe, cigar, or marijuana)	____
Alcohol	I drink less than ten drinks per week and seldom more than two per day	____
Trimness	I am within a few pounds of what I estimate my ideal weight to be	____
Physical Activity	I engage in vigorous physical activity or exercise three hours per week or more	____
Drugs	I rarely use prescription or non-prescription drugs	____
Sleep	I usually get 6-8 hours of sleep daily	____
Breakfast	I eat breakfast regularly	____
Snacking	I seldom eat between meals (exception: raw fruits or vegetables)	____
Diet Additives	I limit the amounts of processed sugar, salt, flour, and chemical additives and preservatives in my diet	____
Blood Pressure	My blood pressure is 120/80 or less (if unknown leave box blank!)	____
For Women Only	For Women Only	____
Breast Examination	I examine myself monthly for lumps	____
Pap Smear	I have one annually	____

upon data regarding the common causes of death from birth to age eighty, and a collaborating study of probable contributing factors. Belloc and Breslow found that the average physical health status of people over age seventy who had none of the risk factors was about the same as those aged thirty-five to forty-four who had five or more of these risk factors. Furthermore, there was a consistent progression toward better health at all ages as the number of good health practices increased.

The scoring of this questionnaire and the other tests are included both as a motivational factor and to determine cumulative points for the "Personal Fitness Profile" included at the end of the chapter. The questionnaire should be presented as it is pictured. The statement of confidentiality is important so that participants will be encouraged to respond accurately.

Test Number 2: Resting Heart Rate

The resting heart rate is a significant indication of improved fitness. The heart rate has a direct relationship to the amount of blood the heart can pump per minute and the reserve capability of the heart for vigorous activities and emergencies. Proper aerobic exercise will cause the resting pulse rate to continue decreasing over a period of time up to a certain point when the ideal metabolic function of an individual is reached. It should be noted however that decreases in resting pulse rate usually require a minimum of twelve weeks training.

The normal adult male has a resting heart rate of around seventy beats per minute. A well conditioned person may have a heart rate below fifty. A female's heart rate is about six beats per minute faster than a male's who is in similar condition. Several studies have found that males with a resting heart rate of over eighty had several times the likelihood of heart attack than men with heart rates under seventy.

There are wide fluctuations in heart rate, even between individuals with equal health and fitness. This should be pointed out to participants to avoid any possible frustration. There are also temporary increases in pulse rate immediately after eating, exercise, changes in position, and during anxiety. For this reason it is important to have subjects in a relaxed state before taking their pulse. It is most convenient to have the subjects sitting. If a table is available, a supine position is alright, but whichever position is used it must be consistent from one testing period to another as the pulse will be slightly lower in a supine position than in a sitting position.

The pulse rate should be felt at the radial artery at the wrist just above the large thumb joint. The pulse should be felt with the tips of the fingers, not the thumb as the thumb has a pulse of its own. A stopwatch should be used and the number of beats felt in thirty seconds should be counted. The total should be multiplied by two to determine the number of beats per minute. This number should then be recorded.

Test Number 3: Resting Blood Pressure

The blood pressure test should also be given while the subject is relaxed and before the other more vigorous tests commence. This is because systolic blood pressure increases with activity. It may also vary slightly from time to time depending on anxiety levels, amount of rest or pressures during the day, and diet. On the average, however, a resting blood pressure will generally indicate the approximate condition of the blood vessels.

Blood pressure measures the pressure of the blood against the arterial walls. There are actually two measurements taken. The first measures the amount of pressure in the artery while the heart muscle is contracting or ejecting blood into the system. This is known as the systolic blood pressure and is represented by the top number in the blood pressure equation. The second measurement measures the pressure in the system in between contractions of the heart. This is known as the diastolic and is the bottom number.

The equipment needed for taking blood pressure includes a sphygmometer and a stethoscope. A blood pressure kit containing these items can be purchased at medical supply stores and many drug stores for less than fifty dollars. Directions are usually included in each kit but can briefly be described as follows.

With the subject in a sitting position with both feet flat on the floor, place the cuff on the arm above the elbow with the arrow pointing to brachial artery on the inside of the elbow. Place the disk of the stethoscope on the artery at that point and pump up the cuff to around one hundred sixty mm/hg (milimeters of mercury) or just until no heart beat sound can be heard. A more accurate way is to simultaneously feel for the radial pulse. When it disappears pump the cuff ten mm/hg higher and stop pumping.

When the dial needle reaches its highest point, slowly release the air pressure so that the needle drops about three mm/hg per second. Listen carefully for the thumping sound of the heart to appear. When it first appears, note the number at which the needle is pointing and continue releasing the pressure. This is the systolic pressure. Now listen carefully for the sound to disappear, which will happen when the pressure in the cuff equals the pressure in the arm. At the point where the sound first disappears or becomes muffled, note the reading on the dial. This is the diastolic blood pressure. At rest, the systolic blood pressure should be eighty or less. Statistically the chances of having a heart attack double when pressures are above these figures. Since the diastolic pressure is somewhat more indicative of vascular condition, this figure should be recorded in the appropriate place on the "Personal Fitness Profile."

If blood pressure at rest is 150/100 or more, it is recommended that the subject not be tested further, although several readings may be necessary to assure accuracy. If the reading remains high, the subject should discreetly be advised to see a physician. Although the fitness leader or technician should be careful not to "practice medicine," he should advise the subject to see a physician, who will recommend a stress test and an exercise and diet regimen. Otherwise, the subject may be sent to his or her doom if a physician recommends medication exclusively and no exercise guidelines, as is sadly sometimes the case.

Test Number 4: Anthropometric Measurements

Direct body measurements are an excellent way to show improvements in both fat loss in overfat individuals and muscular gain in underweight individuals. If a man is interested in increasing muscle size and definition, specific tape measurements of the neck, chest girth, upper arm, forearm, abdomen, upper and lower thigh, and calf muscle should be taken. Most measurements for typical employee fitness programs, however, will be concerned with fat loss. The following measurements should be made with either metric or standard tape measure, and should be recorded to the nearest five-tenths centimeter or one-eighth inch.

Upper Arm - Measure the girth at the widest point between the elbow and the shoulder at the center of the bicep muscle.

Maximal Abdominal Circumference - Measure the maximum abdominal girth between the lowest lateral portion of the rib cage and the iliac crest (the prominent point of the hip bone). Pass the tape around the subject in a horizontal plane. Record.

Hip Circumference - Measure the maximum protrusion of the gluteal muscles (buttocks) at the level of the symphysis pubis (the point where the pubic bones form at the most anterior part of the abdomen or over the crotch area). Pass the tape around the subject in a horizontal plane. Record.

Upper Thigh - Measure the circumference of the thigh at its widest point as above. Record.

In addition to the tape measurements above, skinfold measurements should also be taken. For these measurements a skinfold caliper will be required, and can be purchased for around two hundred dollars for a quality set. The Lang Caliper is recommended as it has a trigger. Skinfold measurements allow actual measurement of the amount of fat at sites where fat usually accumulates.

It is essential that enough practice of the technique of taking skinfold measurements is taken before actual test recordings are made for the program. The skinfold measurement is only valid when done by an experienced tester who can be consistent from one measurement to the next. There are no norms presently available for any of the above measurements. Skinfold measurements should be taken at the following sites:

Pectoral - Pinch a fold of skin with the thumb and forefinger of the left hand. Have the subject flex to find the fat fold and then relax for the measurement. Come down over the top and place calipers underneath fingers and measure fold. The pinch of fat should be taken from a point above the pectoral muscle halfway between the nipple and the axilla or armpit.

Tricep - Using the same technique as for the pectoral measurement, pinch a fold of fat from behind the left arm behind the tricep muscle.

Iliac - Again, using the same technique, pinch a fold of fat from the area just above the iliac crest.

All of the above will be measured in millimeters with standard calipers. These measurements, along with several others, can also be used for determining percentage of body fat with several protocols and should be recorded on two separate forms as appropriate to avoid remeasuring.

Test Number 5: Body Composition

The measurement of body composition refers to ratio of body fat to lean body mass. The determination of one's percentage of body fat and percentage of lean mass (muscle and bone) is the best way to predict an ideal body weight. This method is far superior to the typical height-weight charts used by many insurance companies. An understanding of body composition is also an excellent educational and motivational tool for promoting fat loss programs.

"Ideal" body weight is based on the assumption by health experts that no more than twelve percent of a person's body weight *over and above the percentage of essential fat* should be fat. Since men have about three percent essential body fat, their ideal maximum percentage of body fat should be fifteen percent. Because of the reproductive requirements of women, their essential body fat is about thirteen percent. Their ideal maximum percentage of body fat should be twenty-five percent. These percentages should be considered maximum, and any percentage of fat between the essential level and the maximum level is desired. A long distance male runner, for example, averages five to eight percent body fat.

There are two basic ways that a company can evaluate body composition. The first is anthropometrically and the second is hydrostatically. Anthropometrically determined values are significantly less accurate, but can be used without the costly equipment and space required for hydrostatic weighing. There are several formulas for using anthropometric measurements and all that is required are a calculator, a metric tape, and/or calipers.

The formulas listed are used by various Y.M.C.A. fitness programs throughout the United States.

The first formula is the easiest to compute, although it is more accurate for men than for women. The formula is as follows:
Lean Body Weight (LBW) = 98.42 + (1.082 x body weight (lbs.) - 4.15 x waist girth in inches.
Percent Body Fat = (body weight - lean body weight) x 100 divided by body weight.

A second formula used extensively by Y.M.C.A.s was devised by Zuti and Golding at Kent State in 1972. The formula requires the careful and practiced use of skinfold calipers as described previously. The formula is as follows:
Percent Fat = 8.7075 + .0489309 x waist girth (cm) + .448561 x Pectoral Skinfold (mm) - 6.358583 x right wrist diameter (cm). A conversion table for estimation of percent fat for this protocol is included.

The third formula is for determination of body fat in women and was devised by Wilmore and Benke. A chart for calculating percent of fat using this protocol is on page   .

Another formula for determining body fat in women requires only the skinfold measurement of the iliac and the tricep. The formula is as follows:
Density = 1.0764 - (.00081 x iliac + .00088 x tricep)
Percent Fat = 4.201 divided by Density - 3.813 x 100.

The last method of measurement for determining percentage of fat in women requires a skinfold measurement at the tricep and the scapula, a neck girth, and waist circumference.
Lean Weight = 1.66 + 0.668 x weight (kg) - .158 x scapula (mm) - .081 x tricep (mm) + .555 x neck circumference (cm) - .141 x waist girth.

Percent Fat = weight ÷ total weight (fat weight = total weight less lean weight)

The different measurements are presented so that individuals can choose those that are most effective in yielding a consistent and accurate measurement.

For all methods of determining percent of body fat, including hydrostatic weighing, ideal maximum weight can be calculated as follows:

1. Actual weight x percent fat = fat weight

2. Actual weight x fat weight = lean body mass

3. Ideal maximum body weight for men = lean body mass divided by .85 (for fifteen percent)

4. Ideal maximum body weight for women = lean body mass divided by .75 (for twenty-five percent)

Hydrostatic Weighing

The most accurate means of assessing body fat is hydrostatic weighing. Hydrostatic weighing involves the use of a water tank approximately four feet deep and four feet wide. The tank should have a water heater and should meet the building's fire code. In some cases a hot tub may be used if it is deep enough and a scale can be suspended over it.

A chair can be made out of two inch diameter PVC pipe and should be filled with sand. It need not be complicated but should be made so that a person can sit comfortably in it while submerged for a moment under water. The chair should be bridled to a ring overhead from which an autopsy scale is attached. The scale should be suspended from a ceiling or platform directly over the water tank.

The water temperature should be about thirty-two to thirty-six degrees centigrade. The subject should be placed in the chair so that only the head is above water. When the tester is ready, the subject should expell as much air out of the lungs as possible until the tester can read the weight of the individual while he or she is under water. The weight of the subject under water and the weight of the subject out of the water will be entered into the following equations to determine the percentage of body fat.

Percent Fat = 495 ÷ D - 450 (D represents body density)

D = Weight in Air ÷ (weight in air - weight in water ÷ density of water) - RV + 100 (ml)

For these formulas, the following information is needed:

Weight in Air (determined with standard scale in kilograms)

Weight in Water (determined via underwater weighing in kilograms)

Density of Water = .994 at 36 C (98.6F)

RV = Residual Volume (air left in lungs after expiration): RV = 1.4 liters for male under twenty-five, RV = 1.7 liters for male over twenty-five, RV = 1.0 liters for female under twenty-five, RV = 1.3 liters for female over twenty-five.

Once the subject's percentage of fat is recorded and ideal body weight is calculated at the maximum value, the subject should be educated as to the significance of the information. It should be explained that the ideal maximum weight recommended is for the lean body mass that was currently assessed. If the lean body mass increases via the muscle building exercise program, as is often the case, the ideal maximum weight recommendation can be increased correspondingly. Ideal maximum weight is often what the individual weighed at age eighteen.

Recommendations for fat loss via diet and exercise should be between one and two pounds per week. Although the exercise will play a major role in regulating fat metabolism as well as providing additional caloric expenditure, it is important for the participant to plan a proper diet.

Test Number 6: Vital Capacity and Forced Expiratory Volume

Vital capacity refers to the lungs' capacity for oxygen, and forced expiratory volume in one second measures the lungs' ability to function. Both measurements require the use of a spirometer which can be purchased for around three hundred dollars.

If an individual is within the normal range, as indicated below, on these tests, there will be little change with exercise. People with lower values will usually be asthmatics, smokers, people manifesting allergies, and people with emphysema. Only individuals with extremely poor fitness levels will show improvement otherwise. For these reasons, spirometery might be considered more diagnostic than inspirational and may be considered as an optional test.

Vital Capacity Normal Ranges:

sex	age 16-34	age 35-49	age 50-69
M	2.9-6.1	2.6-5.6	2.1-5.4
F	2.2-4.4	2.0-4.1	1.8-3.8

Forced Expiratory Volume:

M	2.5-4.5	2.1-4.1	1.7-5.2
F	2.1-3.3	1.8-3.0	1.5-2.7

Test Number 7: Cardiorespiratory Endurance (Aerobic Capacity)

Just as cardiovascular training can be considered the "heart" of the fitness program, the evaluation of aerobic or cardiovascular and respiratory capacity is the heart of the fitness testing sequence. Although all of the fitness components are important, cardiovascular and pulmonary efficiency should be the cornerstone of every fitness program.

Maximal oxygen uptake (VO_2) is the maximum amount of oxygen the cardiovascular and respiratory system can deliver to the working muscles. This maximum ability can be increased in unfit individuals but is limited genetically. Once an individual reaches a high degree of fitness, improvements in fitness levels will not significantly increase maximum VO_2, although increased enzyme quality, muscle endurance, and strength (including the heart muscle) will result in higher workload achievement for a given heart rate. (For this reason it is important to record workload, heart rate, and time as well as maximum VO_2).

Tests that measure the ability of the heart, lungs, and blood vessels to transport oxygen to the large working muscles can be divided into "maximal" and "submaximal" tests. A maximal test is one that requires an individual to exercise at such an intensity that a maximum heart rate is attained before the test is ceased. Although such a test is more accurate for determining the maximum amount of oxygen that can be transported, it has several disadvantages for most fitness programs.

The first disadvantage has to do with the increased risk potential of maximal testing. An individual with latent ischemic heart disease is more apt to suffer an infarction during a maximal workload than during a submaximal workload. This consideration will cause many insurance carriers to require the presence of trained medical personnel during such testing.

The second disadvantage of the maximal test is that it requires more time to implement. Tests should be as practical as possible in terms of time and testing expertise, and the maximal test may not be practical in such terms.

The third disadvantage of the maximal test is the unpleasantness associated with such maximal efforts. A participant subjected to such a test is less likely to want to be tested again, and such an attitude defeats the purpose of the test in the first place.

Sub-maximal testing involves workloads at the end of the test that are below maximal exertion. Astrand's calculations of oxygen requirements for given amounts of work, and the linear relationship between heart rate and oxygen uptake, enable maximum oxygen uptake to be predicted from the estimated maximum workload.

The disadvantage of the sub-maximal test is that there is always doubt as to the maximum workload the subject could really have reached. Sub-maximal tests use predicted maximal heart rates based on a formula of two hundred twenty minus age and, although this is accurate enough for determining exercise heart rates, a standard deviation of nine beats a minute can lead to an inaccurate prediction of aerobic capabity.

The best compromise for the measurement is a "near maximal" test. This test will use a treadmill or bicycle ergometer. There should be multiple workloads continuously increased with a minimum of two minutes at each workload. The test should start at a minimal workload for a warm-up and a near maximal capacity should be reached between seven and twelve minutes. Near maximal capacity should be a heart rate equal to two hundred twenty minus age times eighty-five percent. Increases in workloads should be gradual and should be made only after a steady state heart rate has been achieved. (During "steady state" the heart rate will remain constant after two or three minutes at a new workload.)

Although a treadmill has the advantage over the bicycle ergometer in that any individual can be tested regardless of leg strength, the ergometer is less expensive and requires less expertise and time to administer. Therefore, the protocol described below is for a bicycle ergometer.

As an alternative or additional test of cardiorespiratory endurance, the United States Forestry Step Test is presented in Chapter 14. This test is inexpensive and is ideal for self-testing.

Before either test is administered it is important that the symptoms for termination of the test are completely understood by both the subject and the tester. The subject should be advised that he or she should stop the test when any of the symptoms occur and that it is perfectly alright to do so. For measurement purposes, the point at which the test was ceased can be recorded in terms of both time and workload. This measurement will suffice for progress evaluation, although it may not be useful for aerobic capacity determination. The symptoms for termination include:

- dizziness
- angina (pain, usually in chest, shoulder, or arm)
- unusual fatigue
- intolerable pain
- unsteadiness

- mental confusion
- pallor or cyonosis—a sign of insufficient oxygen supply
- rapid breathing or unusually labored breathing
- nausea
- a fall in systolic blood pressure

In addition to the above symptoms, it is also important to communicate with the subject. Sometimes an individual will feel unusual pain but will attempt to hide it. The tester should encourage continual communication during the test by asking the individual how he is feeling at each workload and assuring him that the long-term success of the program depends on a gradual, relatively painful experience.

Bicycle Ergometer Test

A proper bicycle ergometer will cost between four hundred and one thousand dollars. It should have a mechanism for adjusting prescribed workloads for periodic calibration. Workloads are usually measured in kilograms or kiloponds (the force required to lift one kilogram one meter).

The seat on the ergometer should be adjusted so that the leg is slightly bent when fully extended in the downward position. Handlebars should be adjusted so that the subject is slightly leaning forward and is comfortable. The pedaling rate should be synchronized to a metronome at fifty rpm or approximately eighteen kilometers per hour. A blood pressure cuff should be placed on the subject for occasional readings to assure a steady rise in systolic blood pressure and for a pressure-rate score that will be described later.

A stopwatch should be set and the first workload should be set at three hundred kgm/minutes or less so that the first three minutes serves as a gradual warm-up. The pulse rate should be taken for the last fifteen seconds of the third minute. If these two rates are about the same (steady state), then the second workload should be set. This procedure should be repeated for a total of three or four three-minute workloads, and the third minute steady state heart rates should be plotted on a graph.

After the maximum workload has been maintained for the allotted time, the workload should be cut in half and the subject advised to continue pedaling for two minutes. This will provide a sufficient cool-down period.

The chart in the Appendix is used by the Nationwide Y.M.C.A. Cardiovascular Health Program and is based on the calculations of Per-Olof Astrand. Also included is a guide that may be used for setting workloads that was developed by James Havlick of the Inland Empire Y.M.C.A. This should be used as a guide only in case the increased workload stipulated does not result in a steady state.

Astrand's calculation of maximum oxygen uptake in milliliters of oxygen per kilogram of body weight per minute, utilized at maximum functional capacity, is shown. The maximum workload, heart rate, and predicted VO_2 in ml/kg/min should be recorded. The specific rating for age and sex will be used for the "Personal Fitness Profile."

Pulse Rate Index

Since blood pressure readings during the test will be used for possible indications of heart disease and termination of test, a simple systolic reading at the peak workload should be taken for another significant measurement. The systolic blood pressure at peak exercise, times the heart rate at peak exercise divided by one hundred, is the pulse rate index. This measurement can be used for any exercise workload that can be measured and repeated and is recommended by the American Medical Association as an excellent indication of fitness improvement.

Run/Walk Maximum Maximal Oxygen Uptake Predictions

In some instances a fitness director might prefer to do cardiorespiratory testing on a measured track. In this way many people can be tested simultaneously and without any other equipment or facilities. All that is needed is a nearby running track. This type of fitness evaluation is also convenient for self-testing purposes as it can be done by the employee on any track without need of scheduling or company facilities.

The disadvantages of this type of testing should be obvious. The lack of individual monitoring and inability to see fatigue symptoms increases the risk of overuse and heart attack, especially in an unfit population. During group runs it is likely that the competition factor will cause participants to "race" one another, which not only may be unsafe but is also contrary to the objectives of the fitness program. Since individuals may not pace themselves to near maximal or maximal exertion for the entire distance, the accuracy of the maximal oxygen uptake prediction is also poor.

There are two basic ways the group run/walk can be administered. The first requires that a quarter mile track be divided into tenths and marked accordingly. The participant (s) then begin running and run as far as they can for exactly twelve minutes. The distance is recorded and maximal oxygen uptake is predicted using the table. the table.

The second test requires timing a 1.5 mile run at maximal effort. The time the distance was run in is correlated to the tables as above.

A more accurate determination of maximal oxygen uptake for self-evaluation is accomplished with the following protocol. The protocol requires individuals already in better than average condition.

1. Run one-half mile at 120-140 beats per minute heart rate. Record heart rate, time, and distance.

2. Rest and repeat at 150-170 beats per minute heart rate and record as above.

3. Run at maximum effort for three to six minutes, sprinting at the finish. Take a ten second pulse count and record "maximal heart rate" in beats per minute.

4. Determine the oxygen cost for running at the two sub-maximal paces from the chart below.

5. Using the graph and tables for the bicycle ergometer test, plot the two sub-maximal heart rates and the maximal heart rate, and draw a horizontal line through the maximal heart rate.

6. Drop the line from the intersection of the sub-maximal rates with the maximal heart rate to find maximal oxygen uptake.

7. Add five to ten percent to allow for curve in linear relationship between oxygen utilization and heart rate.

Steady State O_2 Cost of Running

MPH	½ Mile	Mile Pace	ml/kg/min
6	5:00	10:00	33.3
7	4:17	8:34	39.4
7.5	4:00	8:00	42.4
8.	3:45	7:30	45.6
8.5	3:32	7.04	48.6
9.	3:20	6:40	51.8
9.5	3:10	6:20	55.1
10.	3:00	6:00	58.2
10.5	2.52	5:44	61.5
11.	2:44	5:28	64.8
11.5	2:37	5:14	68.1
12.	2:30	5:00	71.5
12.5	2:24	4:48	74.9
13.	2:18	4:36	78.4
13.5	2:09	4:18	86.5

Test Number 8: Recovery Index

Another measurement of cardiovascular fitness has to do with the ability to recover after strenuous exercise. The more rapidly the heart rate and respiration return to a resting rate, the more fit an individual is.

The protocol for measuring the recovery rate is designed for use with the bicycle ergometer. At the end of the two minute cool-down at one-half workload intensity, the subject should sit quietly for fifteen seconds. Immediately following the fifteen seconds rest, the heart rate should then be counted for one full minute.

The recovery index is obtained by dividing the *resting pulse rate* before the test by the post-exercise one minute recovery pulse rate. The quotient will result in the percentage of recovery. The following rating can be used.

85-100% = excellent
75-84%   = good
66-74%   = average

Test Number 9: Flexibility

Trunk flexion is one of the most appropriate and easily administered tests of flexibility for both men and women. This test will measure the flexibility of the torso and hamstrings. The importance of flexibility in these areas cannot be overemphasized, as the majority of lower back problems as well as many athletic injuries result from inadequate flexibility.

This test is also an excellent motivator as gains in flexibility occur rapidly with training. Such a "minor success" often can motivate participants to try harder to improve more difficult measurements.

The measurement is made with the subject sitting on the floor or table with legs outstretched at shoulder width. A tape measure is stretched between the legs with the one inch mark toward the crotch so that the fifteen inch mark is on a line with the heels of the foot (not the shoe). The subject should then reach forward as far as possible, keeping both knees flat on the surface. A score of fifteen means the subject has "touched his or her toes," thirteen inches means two inches short of toes, and seventeen inches means two inches beyond the toes.

Although the above method works fine, especially for self-testing, a more permanent method should be devised. One way is to simply mark the appropriate measurements on a table or bench. Another is to make a "flexometer." This can be simply made as follows:

Start with a two by five foot masonite or plywood board, sanded and finished. Groove a slot at one end in the center of the board about one inch wide and thirty-six inches long. Alongside the groove inlay a yardstick. On a line even with the fifteen inch mark, attach heel blocks at approximately shoulder width with a person sitting on the board with the feet pointing toward the grooved end. Finally, attach a block of wood five to six inches square, perpendicular to a 7/8 inch wide by eight inch long block of wood that will fit and slide into the groove.

With this device, the subject pushes the block with hands outstretched as far as possible, and the reading can be made at the point where the nearest edge of the block meets the rule. It is important that the subject be allowed three practice warm-ups and keeps knees flat. The tester may have to hold the knees down to assure an accurate reading.

The following ratings can be used:

Men:		Women:	
Excellent	22-23 inches	Excellent	24-27 inches
Good	20-21 inches	Good	21-23 inches
Average	14-18 inches	Average	16-20 inches
Fair	12-13 inches	Fair	13-16 inches

Test Number 9: Muscular Strength

Although there are many tests for measuring muscular strength, it is difficult to choose one that men and women of all ages and fitness levels can do without undue difficulty. For this reason, a grip strength test is often used. This requires the purchase of a hand dynomometer at a cost of around one hundred dollars. The grip strength correlates about twenty-five percent of total body strength but usually improves as total body strength improves. The reading is usually in kilograms.

In order to perform the test, the subject must forcefully and suddenly squeeze the dynomometer. The highest reading will be used for the score. Several attempts should be allowed.

The test can be rated as follows:

Men:		Women:	
Excellent	66-70	Excellent	37-40
Good	58-62	Good	29-36
Average	46-54	Average	22-27
Fair	38-42	Fair	17-21
Poor	30-34	Poor	13-16

Test Number 10: Muscular Endurance

Three tests have been chosen for measuring muscular endurance. They include bent knee sit-ups, the bench press, and the hanging arm flexion.

For the sit-up test, have the subject lie on his or her back with knees bent so that heels are about one foot from the buttocks. The subject's feet should be held down. The subject's hands should be clasped behind the head. A stopwatch should be started as the individual commences sitting up as many times as possible so that the elbows touch the knees. The test ends at exactly one minute and the number of sit-ups accomplished are recorded.

Sit-Up Rating:

Excellent	35 +		Average	20-29
Good	30-34		Fair	15-19

Bench Press

The bench press requires a standard bench press and a barbell with fifty-five pounds which can be purchased for around one hundred dollars. After instructions and a demonstration of the proper bench press technique by the fitness director or tester, the subject lies on his or her back and receives the barbell in a flexed elbow position. The subject then extends the elbows to press the barbell upward until the elbows are extended and returns the barbell to the chest position as many times as possible without resting between presses.

For the women's test thirty-five pounds of weight should be used. For the men's test fifty-five pounds should be used. The ratings below apply to these weights.

Excellent	37-46 times		Fair	5-11 times
Good	24-36 times		Poor	0-4 times
Average	12-23 times			

Hanging Arm Flexion

The third test alternative for muscular endurance merely requires a stopwatch and a chinning bar. The subject should hang from the bar with the chin just over the bar and the palms facing outward. The rating is as follows:

Men:		Women:	
Excellent	2:00	Excellent	1:30 - 1:59
Good	1:30 - 1:59	Good	45 - 1:15
Average	1:15 - 1:29	Average	30 - 45

After completion of the tests, all scores should be recorded on a form that can be permanently filed and given to the participant. In this way the participant will have all the information for "taking the mystery" away from test results, and the company will also have the results for aggregate evaluations, program adjustments, and in case the participant loses his or her scores.

The scores applicable should also be charted on a "Personal Fitness Profile." Such a profile will show an overall picture of the individual's fitness level and will make it easier to observe fitness improvements. The fitness profile includes the major evaluations. Different colors should be used to block in the area beneath the total point score.

In addition to the ten evaluations, one final "evaluation" should be made at the completion of the tests and after everyone has participated in the fitness testing experience. This final test is merely a written estimate of the participant's perceived level of fitness. The question should be handed out, confidentially answered, and collected. The question should be phrased as follows:

HOW PHYSICALLY FIT DO YOU FEEL AT THE PRESENT?
Unfit   below average   average   above average   very fit

This is an important self-evaluation because it acknowledges the "unmeasurable" benefits of fitness, i.e., "feeling better." Furthermore, the NASA study showed a high correlation between perceived levels of fitness and actual fitness levels. By administering the question at the end of the program, it allows people to reflect on their previous attempts at the evaluations and climaxes the testing with, perhaps, the most important consideration.

Blood Chemistry

Another tool is blood chemistry analysis, including such measurements as HDL/cholesterol and total cholesterol. To be optimally effective, however, blood samples should be taken once a week for three weeks, and averaged.

10

ORGANIZING THE OPERATION

The components of selling, developing, implementing, and evaluating an employee fitness program have been presented. With the information contained in the previous chapters, the reader should have a thorough understanding of the many dimensions of employee fitness. To further assist the individual who is prepared to take action in implementing a program, this chapter will consolidate the many considerations into an operational blueprint.

MANAGEMENT BY OBJECTIVES

A prerequisite to any successful employee fitness program is the application of sound managerial principles. The first and foremost principle is to maintain an awareness of the goals and objectives of the program. These objectives should be both tangible and intangible. Tangible objectives should include:

- measurable improvements in aggregate fitness levels based on individual fitness measurements described in Chapter 9
- short- and long-term decreases in absenteeism
- reduced employee turnover
- short- and long-term reductions in medical costs and compensation
- increased working longevity of key employees (long-term)
- possible decreases in medical insurance premiums
- increased work productivity or measurable improvement in quality of service

Intangible objectives should include:

- improved employee morale
- employees with a better attitude toward work and play
- employees with a happier home life
- employees who can handle stress better
- employees who get along better with fellow workers and management

Such a list of objectives should be published and reviewed regularly by all persons involved in managing and implementing the program. When an organization loses sight of its basic objectives, its programs lose their intrinsic meaning and the flow of energy becomes stifled by systematic procedure. Many management tasks fail when such basic objectives are forgotten, but a physical fitness program is especially vulnerable.

Just as there should be a review of the long and short-term goals of the program, there should also be a continual review of the objectives of program management. These objectives should include:

1. a strong managerial commitment to the program

2. a well-planned and organized operation

3. a creative facility and program

4. an obligation to experiment and change when appropriate

5. a continual awareness of expansion potential and feasibility

6. continual evaluation of all aspects of the program

7. continual search for new motivational techniques

8. continual marketing to create a demand for the program from uninvolved employees

9. efficient record keeping

10. good communication among various levels within the organization

11. a consistent philosophy of exercise and fundamental principles of wellness

12. a commitment to making the program as much fun as possible

13. a commitment to the priority that employees are people

1. A strong managerial commitment to the physical fitness program is essential if a high level of participation at the sub-management level is desired. Not only must management maintain a commitment to the program objectives and the management objectives, but management personnel should be visibly active in the program as well. As soon as employees realize that their superiors are not

exercising and participating in the educational seminars they will begin to react with apathy and even defensiveness themselves. Failure of management to participate in an employee fitness program is a sure way to stifle widespread participation.

2. A well-planned and organized operation should remain an important objective throughout the life of the program. The investment, responsibilities, and rewards of a fitness program are no less deserving of such consideration than the business itself. Constant attention to details and efficiency will produce pride and faith in the fitness program and will increase the possibilities of long-term success.

3. Every fitness program should have its own degree of sparkle and excitement. The decor of the facilities, musical accompaniment to exercise, creative incentives and procedures, and pleasant reminders about health habits on bulletin boards all add to the enjoyability and subsequent success of a fitness program.

4. An obligation to experiment and change a procedure when appropriate should be an ongoing objective of every fitness program director. New approaches might work where old approaches didn't. Monotony can be avoided with a new routine, different music, or new motivational techniques. Scheduling and exercise days can be modified. Exercise alternatives can be substituted. Everyone involved should be willing to experiment.

5. Management should also be continually aware of expansion possibilities. The goal of a program is to get as many employees involved in healthy behavior as possible, and any opportunity that makes this possible should be considered.

6. A continual evaluation of all aspects of the fitness program will assure that an optimal effort is being made to get people fit. If a program isn't working there is usually a reason for it, but if it is not known for sure that it is not working, the failures will quietly reach a point of no return. Employee fitness programs are a new concept and every aspect of the programs should be continually scrutinized for ways to improve. Furthermore, each group of employees is unique and what works for one group may not be effective for another. Continued evaluation and follow-up of individual fitness improvements is also an important motivational device, as was discussed in the previous chapter.

7. A continual search for new motivational techniques is also applicable to the unique needs of a group of participants. Behavior modification and health psychology are just beginning to understand what motivates people to practice healthy habits. As more informa-

tion emerges, managers of a fitness program should be prepared to try the new ideas.

8. As capabilities for facility expansion increase the desire for more participants should also increase. By maintaining a market plan that creates a demand for the fitness program from those employees who are uninvolved, more people can be admitted to the program as soon as facilities are expanded. Maintaining the demand from non-participants also encourages current participants to stay in a program, especially if they have to go to the end of a waiting list once they withdraw from the program.

9. Efficient record keeping is the foundation of the evaluation objective. Attendance records, fitness scores, scheduling, educational programming, and progress reports are all dependent on efficient record keeping. Everyone involved in managing the program should appreciate the importance of this, not only for the company but for the sake of the entire employee fitness movement.

10. Good communication among various levels within the organization will enforce the "happy people" concept. Sub-management employees will continue to feel that the program is theirs as well as management's. The fitness program will continue to provide inter-relations that will increase job satisfaction. Improvements and needs can be more directly identified if communication remains open between participants and program management.

11. The continual programming of education is another objective that management should not forget. A permanent change in health behavior can only result from an increase in wisdom, and wisdom is the experiential application of information. Employees must have the opportunity to receive this information. They should understand what is happening to the body and its systems during exercise. They should understand why certain foods are harmful. They should understand the causes of obesity, hypoglycemia, heart disease, and cancer. They should understand the relationship between a happy life and a healthy life. Such continual education may be the only way to affect a permanent change in lifestyle.

12. A consistent philosophy of exercise and fundamental principles of well-being will provide a foundation for this education. There are many contradictory statements about exercise, nutrition, and other health care considerations that can confuse and overwhelm an individual. If proper statements regarding these subjects are consistently espoused and expressed by program managers the confusion can be diminished. With this consistency employees will not tend to doubt the validity of the program. There are enough

exercise and nutritional principles that are generally recognized as accurate that adhering to such consistent education and philosophy should not be difficult.

13. With all the objectives, responsibilities, efficiency reports, and other efforts necessary to implement a successful fitness program, it may be easy for program managers and leaders to omit a commitment to having fun with the program. There is no meaning to a fitness program if it cannot be related somehow to play. Furthermore, people will be more likely to continue participating if there is an element of fun that pervades the atmosphere.

14. Similarly, it is important that exercise leaders and program managers remember that program participants are not just objects to be measured for improvements in productivity and efficiency. Participants are people and every attempt should be made to keep the "people perspective" in perspective!

DEVELOPMENTAL METHODOLOGY

Once a program has been sold and a comprehensive specific needs analysis has been initially completed, the fitness director can begin the steps necessary for actual program development. The many considerations that must be addressed can be put into perspective by listing them and describing the actions that should be taken. Although there will be some considerations that will be unique to a particular company, the major developmental functions are listed and described below.

- Begin a search for qualified staffing
- Develop and publish a policy statement regarding the program
- Initiate an awareness campaign
- Locate and equip the exercise facilities
- Specify and describe specific program (s)
- Select a pilot group
- Prepare forms and filing system
- Commence medical screening where appropriate
- Proceed with initial fitness testing for all participants
- Schedule participants into program

1. The selection of a director for the fitness program is one of the first actions that should be taken. His or her expertise can then be used to develop the program. Guidelines have already been presented for the selection of qualified personnel.

2. The first action of the fitness director should be to prepare a

comprehensive policy statement about the program. The statement should be prepared in cooperation with company management and should be published for review by all employees. The policy statement should include the following information:

a. the purpose of the fitness program

b. a brief description of the program

c. an explanation of the availability of the program

d. an introduction to the leadership personnel

e. a statement about the confidentiality of fitness evaluations

The wording of the "purpose" section of the policy should be carefully constructed. The program should appear to be a response to employee desires as opposed to being a paternal action or managerial mandate. The purpose should be described as an intention to help employees achieve a fitness level which will afford them a more enjoyable work life, a more enjoyable private life, and a reduction in illness and premature retirement.

In the program description it should be emphasized that participants should attempt to improve their individual fitness levels without competing with one another. It should also be mentioned that current fitness levels or improvement levels during the program will have no negative influence on job security, although improved fitness levels might have a positive influence.

3. Following the publication of the policy statement a larger scale promotional campaign should be developed. The campaign should be a "soft sell" approach to making employees aware of the benefits of proper exercise. This campaign can be conducted with creative posters, occasional lectures, and announcements about community fitness activities. A fitness newsletter can be started or a subscription to one of the commercial fitness letters (see Appendix) can be distributed. This awareness campaign should exist for at least a month before the actual program begins.

4. Based on the surveys and specific needs analysis, the director should be able to choose the appropriate type of program for the employees. With this information he or she will be able to select an appropriate facility. The following outline will summarize the considerations for a facility:

a. The proper size should be based on type of program and capacity at peak use.

b. If an exercise room is used it should be adequately ventilated, and the temperature should be between sixty and seventy degrees. Where possible, wall-to-wall carpeting, background music, and attractive decor should be provided. A bulletin board should be established to post information relative to health and exercise.

c. Adequate locker room, dressing area, and shower facilities should be provided if possible. Arrangements should be made for these areas, as well as the exercise areas, to be kept in top hygenic condition for health as well as motivational purposes.

d. Special equipment should be purchased if required. The selection of equipment should be made by the fitness director who is knowledgeable about equipment quality. If a group exercise program is implemented, floor mats and pacing clocks should be purchased. If possible, towels, soap, and uniforms should be provided to participants. This will add to the program's convenience and sophistication.

e. The facility should include a consideration of emergency situations. Such considerations include an expedient system of securing help, e.g., access to phones or switchboard, trained personnel available at all times during classes, posters describing emergency procedures, and oxygen equipment (optional).

5. After the appropriate facilities are established, a specific format for the fitness programs to be implemented should be published for the exercise leaders. This will assure a consistency in the exercise sessions and will assure that all the proper components are being accomplished. The format should include directions for new participant orientation and a step-by-step description of the exercise session that includes:

a. the purpose of each particular exercise from the warm-up to the cool-down

b. a description of how each exercise should be done

c. a list of precautions applicable to each exercise

d. the time frame and progressions allotted for each exercise

e. a description of important leadership considerations applicable to each exercise.

A format can be developed for a circuit training program that is being supervised by a fitness leader. In those instances where facilities are not supervised, portions of the format can be posted near the exercise stations for the participant to read. Also included in the format is a "tickler list" that an instructor can establish for remembering those pieces of information that will be useful in the education of the participant.

6. The next step is to select a pilot group to begin the program. By limiting initial enrollment to a smaller group, it will be easier to concentrate on presenting an efficient program. If the original participants are highly motivated, the results of the pilot program can often bring forth a larger commitment to a program from management.

Selection of the initial participants can be on a first come, first served basis, a random or lottery selection, or a selection of a single department or group of executives. In any case it is wise to include some top management and union personnel. Initial exclusion from the program because of limited enrollment may also serve to create a demand for the program from non-participants. A minimum attendance should be required if a person is to remain in the program.

7. Before prospective participants are medically screened and tested for fitness levels, an efficient and complete record keeping system should be established. Forms will be needed for individual fitness progress records, for nutritional evaluations, testing protocols and periodic fitness evaluations, attendance records, liability releases (informed consents to participate), and fitness profiles. Although some of these forms are contained in the Appendix, a fitness director may have his or her own preference in designing the forms. Once the forms are all prepared, an efficient system of completing the forms and filing them should be developed. Charts used for individual fitness progress can be stored in paper slots so participants will not lose them.

8. The question of medical screening may be the most controversial of all program considerations. The American Heart Association Committee on Exercise recommends that "before beginning an exercise program that will demand a major increase in physical activity, an individual should be evaluated by his physician. Persons with increased risk factors should undergo exercise stress testing..."

The American Medical Association's Committee on Exercise and the President's Council on Physical Fitness and Sports states that "All candidates for a company sponsored physical fitness program should obtain medical clearance for physical activity. In some instances, modified exercise programs will be recommended based on medical evaluation. Results of the participant's progress in the exercise program should be sent to the medical director on a periodic schedule."

The usual recommendation is that prior to participating in an exercise class, a person should obtain a signed statement from a physician, clearing him for the program and specifying any limitations. Unfortunately this recommendation is not supported by a large professional consensus. Exercise testing in apparently healthy individuals under the age of thirty-five is not likely to disclose more than one case in a hundred that reveals latent ischemic heart disease (any impairment to the transfer of oxygen). At any age group there is a significant percentage of false positive readings that can lead to unnecessary restrictions that are more harmful than helpful.

One of the objectives of fitness programs is to give an individual responsibility for his health and take it away from the medical profession to some degree. According to an article in the *British Columbia Medical Journal*, the authors of an investigation into alternatives for screening high risk adults concluded that "Although many physicians deem regular physical examinations to be important, the necessity and feasibility of having all apparently healthy individuals have a complete medical check before beginning a physical activity program must be questioned."

The article continues, "Extensive pre-exercise evaluation has its scientific and clinical merits....However, such procedures tend to be time-consuming, expensive, and of questionable necessity for many adults. Furthermore, the imposition of pre-exercise medical screening may deter some adults from participating, although prevailing medical opinion holds that most adults do need regular exercise."

A leading Canadian cardiologist, Dr. G.R. Cumming, also addresses the advantages and disadvantages of pre-program exercise electrocardiography and medical screening requirements. He makes the following conclusions in an article titled, "Exercise E.C.G. Tests Prior to Exercise Programs in Well Persons:"

> Exercise testing in well persons for precise exercise prescription is theoretically sound, but may cause more problems than it solves.
> The exercise electrocardiogram has serious limitations as a diagnostic and prognostic test. Concern over exercise E.C.G. changes in well persons can lead to unnecessary restrictions for subjects capable of exercising, and can lead to anxiety and iatrogenic disease (diseases caused by the medical treatment, unnecessary medical consultation, further investigation, and ineffective therapy). A false sense of security may follow a normal E.C.G. test.
> Exercise electrocardiography is not recommended to the public or to the professions dealing with health, exercise, sports, and recreation as a useful general screening procedure to safeguard the health of asymptomatic persons wishing to increase their physical activity. This applies to all age groups. Its main use should be for the safe conduct of exercise tests.

If large populations of individuals are to be encouraged to participate in physical activity, the anxiety, apprehension, inconvenience, and cost associated with medical clearances for exercise will have to be eliminated. The best way to eliminate these barriers is to eliminate the perceived need and reliance on the medical profession. The best safeguard for the unfit people is a proper understanding of exercise and wellness principles. Such persons should enter a fitness program gradually. They should exercise at an intensity that is proper and should slow down for any symptoms, e.g., shortness of breath, dizziness, or pain. Proper fitness program leadership, policy, and instructional supervision should be used in combination with the non-physician-administered tests for most individuals, instead of traditional medical screening and exercise stress tests. Stress tests may be used for individuals displaying multiple risk factors, but only for exercise prescriptions—not to determine if participation is possible.

9. Once the medical screening aspects have been considered, the next step is to initiate fitness testing for each of the participants. The announcement of the testing should emphasize that scores are only important in terms of measuring progress. People should look forward to being evaluated without apprehension or competitive anxiety. The testing protocol should be well-organized and well-recorded. The participant should leave the testing area with an increased awareness of fitness principles and should be motivated to improve.

10. The final developmental step is to schedule participants into the program. If time is not allotted during working hours, facilities should be made available during morning and afternoon breaks, during the lunch hour (s), and before and after working hours. If there is an imbalance in the number of people involved in the program at the various shifts, and space and supervision are limited, it may not be possible for employees to use the various times totally at random. In such cases schedules can be devised based on seniority, lottery, and alphabet ranking.

If the program is to be available on company time, schedules will have to consider work responsibilities. Obviously the business cannot shut down to facilitate the fitness program. Department supervisors should determine how many people can leave an area at what time. In some cases it may be necessary for employees to double up on duties while someone is exercising.

Although the scheduling will require careful planning and extremely organized implementation, it should not become a hassle for employees to exercise. If one employee wants to trade times with another, it should be allowed. If work responsibilities will not be jeopardized, employees should be allowed to use the facility at their own time preference as long as crowding does not occur.

MAINTENANCE AND GROWTH

Successful maintenance and growth of an employee fitness program will depend on the administration of the following ten functions:

- staff assessment meetings
- fitness testing follow-up
- continual motivational campaigns
- program alternative development
- educational activities
- demand stimulation
- program expansion
- public relations outside company
- reports to management
- contribution to national effort

1. The importance of proper program management and leadership has been emphasized. To assure that a high quality of supervision is maintained, regular staff assessment meetings should be scheduled. Via observation and employee criticism reports, strengths and weaknessess of supervision and program direction should be analyzed and adjustments made. Furthermore, the staff should be required to maintain their own fitness requirements and should be continually expanding their own education.

2. One of the most common failures of exercise programs is a lack of follow-up. Programs often start with basic fitness measurements to motivate individuals, but fail to continue with progress measurements. Fitness re-evaluations should be scheduled for each employee at least once every three months and preferably monthly. Employees will look forward to their improvements and will try harder when they know they will be measured soon. Also, the progress is important for assessment of the program's success.

3. Motivation to continue fitness programs will vary from person to person and will even change for a single person. If people are to be expected to remain with a program and not just be a starter, a continuous motivational campaign employing all of the concepts described above is imperative.

4. Just as motivational efforts should be varied and changing, it is also important for the program itself to be varied. Any good exercise program can become monotonous if it does not constantly change. In group programs different exercises can be used, different music played, or the sequences changed. Members of the group can occasionally lead exercises. Various sports and games can be substituted. Competitive sports can be modified to minimize competition and maximize proper exercise. A good fitness director will know how to develop program alternatives within the scope of the facilities.

5. The most essential component in permanently changing life-style behavior is education. Motivational gimmicks and charismatic leadership can only hold a person's interest for so long. A permanent change must come from an intrinsic understanding of the value of the changes. This understanding comes from the experience and knowledge that relates health and happiness to the behavior modifications. A program of ongoing education must be implemented. The program might include:

a. informative talks on some aspect of physical fitness as part of the exercise sessions

b. continuously updated bulletin board

c. lecture programs with guest speakers

d. newsletters

e. posters

f. the creation of a fitness library

6. The continued success of a business is based on marketing activities that continually create a demand for the product or services. The success of a fitness program is similar. The more employees who participate in the program, the higher will be the economic benefits to the company. By continually creating a demand through the existence of a good program and the application of appropriate marketing techniques, a demand can eventually be created for the program that will gradually draw in more employees.

7. As demand increases for the program, there must be a capability to meet the demand. Program directors should begin planning for program expansion as the first signs of a successful program appear. Just as the program was initially sold to management, a request for expansion of facilities must be sold. Details about facilities, costs, additional equipment, personnel, and potential participants will have to be analyzed. Expansion of the program should not be delayed, or prospective participants may lose interest; cur-

rent facilities should not be crammed, or everyone may lose interest.

8. The successful growth of a fitness program is not just related to the increased health of the employees. A successful fitness program that is highly visible can be used as a public relations tool. It can be used to recruit talented personnel. It can be used to develop a company image that might increase sales. It can put a company in good standing with communities. Company facilities can be used for conferences and community programs. Management should make every effort to capitalize on the fitness program. The improvement of public relations will bring added benefits to the company and will also further motivate employees by creating a sense of pride in their organization.

9. Since the top management, owners, or Board of Directors are ultimately responsible for the continuation of an employee fitness program, they should remain informed about the program's progress. An official system for reporting will acknowledge respect for their authority and interest in the program, and will provide an incentive for the staff to maintain a well-planned program with specific objectives for improvement.

10. As employee fitness programs emerge throughout the nation, and inspirational information and evidence become available to all, existing fitness programs will take pride in their pioneering efforts. As general acceptance of employee fitness prevails there will be less of a chance that a program will collapse because of a change in management. There will be less of a chance that management will have misgivings about the long range benefits if others all around are doing the same. It will take less courage for employees and employers to make decisions about employee fitness if it becomes commonplace.

Any effort to contribute to the national effort of health maintenance programs will be an effort to maintain one's own program. Good records should be kept and evidence of improvement should be sent to the President's Council on Physical Fitness and Sports and the American Association of Fitness Directors in Business and Industry. Newspapers and professional magazines should receive articles about the program's benefits. Radio announcements can be used to spread the word. Community projects that use the success of the program to motivate the community into healthy lifestyles can also be implemented.

A fitness director thus has many roles in developing and maintaining a successful fitness program. By organizing his goals and objectives and following the above operational methodology, he or she can be proud of having achieved a most rewarding career.

PART THREE: ORGANIZING FITNESS PROGRAMS IN THE COMMUNITY

11

FITNESS IN THE COMMUNITY

Many companies have recognized the importance of an image that depicts a company that is sincerely concerned with the welfare of its consumer community. This image is becoming increasingly important as the integrity of business comes under more scrutiny. One of the best ways for a company to demonstrate its concern is to participate in organizing health and fitness programs for children, seniors, housewives, and other members of the community.

There is much evidence to support the lucrative potential for such an image. This is why product advertising often depicts the healthy outdoor life. This is why the "we care" approach is inherent in a company's public relations. If a consumer is to trust a company's product or service, he or she must believe that the company is, at least, interested in his or her well-being.

Organizing fitness programs in the community also augments the employee's sense of job satisfaction. A community fitness program is a logical extension of the employee fitness program. Such programs increase opportunities for an employee's family to join in a healthy lifestyle. Opportunities for fitness activities outside the workplace enhance the employee's own fitness program. The employee can also take pride in knowing that his company is making a meaningful contribution to the society in which he lives.

THE "HEALTH CARE" RIP OFF

Before an effective health and fitness program can be developed within the community, the members of the community must be responsive to the need for such programs. Unfortunately, the average citizen has been somewhat duped into thinking that everything possible is being done already in the field of health care. Most communities have a variety of health care agencies, and miraculous drugs and surgery techniques are regularly brought to public attention. The health care statisticians continue to report significant improvements in American life expectancy and decreases in heart disease. If a person is concerned about improved health care, he merely needs to buy a better insurance policy to alleviate the worries, or so he is led to believe.

The community's misconceptions about the need for health programs involves misinformation as well as a lack of information. The phrase "health care" programs are actually "disease care" programs. Those that are oriented toward actual health care usually include programs that emphasize the prevention of communicable disease and in some cases prenatal care. Rare are the programs that emphasize the prevention of heart and lung disease, cancers, obesity, diabetes, and acute depression.

There is also misinformation with regard to the actual state of America's health. One of the great misinterpretations of health statistics is that the health care professionals have done much to improve life expectancy. In fact, the life expectancy for adults has not increased significantly. Although life expectancy from birth has increased twenty-five years since 1900, life expectancy from age fifteen is about the same now as it was then, if maternal mortality is subtracted. A great deal has been done to reduce infant and maternal mortality, but reductions in death by communicable disease has been more than offset by deaths that are diseases of lifestyle. The average age of death of the signers of the Declaration of Independence is similar to the male adult's average age at death today.

Not only has there not been a significant increase in life span as is often believed, but the United States, with all its medical specialization and technology, fares poorly in comparisons of world health status. According to the 1976 *Statistical Abstract of the United States*, the United States ranks twenty-third in life expectancy at birth for males and eighth for life expectancy of females. Even with regard to infant mortality, the United States ranks sixteenth, with almost twice the infant deaths of Sweden.

Misconceptions regarding actual health status exist because of an overconfidence in the health care profession. This overconfidence is exemplified in many ways. Early in 1976 a congressional subcommittee estimated the number of unnecessary operations at nearly 2.5 million a year, at a monetary cost of more than 3.5

billion dollars and at a human cost of twelve thousand deaths. A *New York Times* article reached a similar conclusion. According to cardiologist Julia Whitacker, ninety percent of all bypass operations are unnecessary. Without a lifestyle change patients will be back in the same condition in several years, but fifty thousand dollars poorer.

More important than overconfidence in the medical profession is the reason for the overconfidence. The average citizen has become resigned to passivity in the area of health care. He has come to expect that things will be taken care of by government or the medical profession, or some energetic radical who would not tolerate too great an inadequacy. After all, this is how medical research, water purification, milk pasteurization, immunization and sanitation, and other progressive health measures have come about.

The failure to intervene actively on one's own behalf is what has given government and the medical profession the awesome capability to waste money and provide insignificant health care measures. It should be realized that more physicians, medical facilities, and technologies have little to do with the major plagues to human health and happiness that exist today. Each American is paying almost seven hundred dollars per year for "health care." Although this money may result in the economic or political gain for its recipients, too much of this cost has too little effect on the health and well-being of its payers. The protection of health and well-being can only result from personal intervention into lifestyle.

Any successful intervention into living, however, requires information upon which to act. The information must also be processed in such a way as to make it functional and applicable to the objective. This process, or education, is essential for a community that becomes aware of the need for improved health maintenance. It is here, within the existing educational process, where the basic cause of the failure to assume responsibility for health care can be found. Adequate health education does not exist. Educational priorities are influenced politically, not morally.

The political influence on health education, or the lack of it, should be understood by every adult within a community if a successful community fitness program is to be expected. Although little is ever gained by pointing fingers at villains, an exposure of inadequacies might at least end dependence on them.

First of all, it should be realized that physicians control the majority of information that is typically channeled into health education. This presents a problem because the majority of physicians are not particularly interested in educating the public to prevent disease or cut health costs. Most physicians are not involved in promoting meaningful health education because the financial, emotional, and intellectual rewards of carrying out health education programs are negligible for most physicians. It is more rewarding to practice acute, curative medicine.

It is also important to note that the majority of physicians are not knowledgeable about those considerations most vital to community health education. Very few medical schools teach exercise physiology or nutrition. Very few teach the importance of patient health education and responsibility. In the growing age of medical specialization, there is no specialty in health maintenance or disease prevention. Perhaps such a specialty is a threat to job security in the profession.

The influence of the medical profession is also projected upon health educators themselves. The majority of public health schools still do not provide sufficient information about diseases linked to modern lifestyle. The author has interviewed many public health educators who could not properly define blood pressure, discuss basic nutritional principles, or describe the importance of regular physical activity. In many instances the individuals were in need of health education themselves.

The medical community is also largely in control of where taxpayer money for health care services goes. In 1974, $1.78 billion dollars was allocated for health related research. Most of the money was allocated for biomedical research directed toward improving the physician's ability to treat and cure. Of the remainder, seventy million dollars was expended to improve the capability of the medical care delivery system.

In 1972, Congress authorized thirty centers to test and apply existing knowledge toward the prevention of disease. Today there are only five in existence. Of these five, only two are involved with health education and lifestyle intervention relating to blood pressure, smoking, and cholesterol; and these two are losing funding. The other three relate to drug management for hypertension, heart disease, and bypass operations. None of them relate to physical activity.

In 1976, government responded to the outcry for health maintenance programs with Public Law 94-317, the "Health Information and Health Promotion Act of 1976." In Section 1703, "Community Programs," the law states that the Secretary of Health is authorized to "conduct and support new and innovative programs in health information and promotion, preventive health services, and education in the appropriate use of health care, and support demonstration and training programs in various settings that focus on objectives which are measurable and emphasize the prevention or moderation of illness or accidents that appear controllable through individual knowledge and behavior..."

In 1977, ten million dollars was authorized for such programs and zero dollars appropriated. In 1979, seventeen million dollars was authorized and 1.2 million dollars appropriated, most of which was used to set up administrative offices.

Another law, also passed to promote health and decrease health care costs, is similarly under the control of the traditional medical community. The "National Health Planning and Resources Development Act of 1974," Public Law 93-641, was intended to define national priorities and guidelines for health planning. It also provided for the establishment of area planning agencies responsible for developing priorities and implementing programs for meeting objectives.

Although participation in these agencies is opened to members of the general public, the potential threat of mandates that might stifle traditional medical expenditures prompted the "infiltration" of physicians into the official agency affairs. The physicians, being the most active participants on the various councils, managed to protect vested interests in many instances. In other instances a quagmire of legalities and other policy challenges have impeded any effective action.

Among possible priorities, two have received little more than lip service in most of the planning areas. These relate to preventive services and health education within the community:

● The promotion of activities for the prevention of disease, including studies of nutritional and environmental factors affecting health and the provision of preventive health care services.

● The development of effective methods of educating the general public concerning proper personal (including preventative) health care methods for effective use of available health services.

It must be remembered that inaction relating to such priorities cannot be blamed on the medical profession, but on the lack of awareness and apathy of the community. The medical community is looking after its interests. The general population should look after its own welfare as well.

One reason why advocacy for prevention has come mainly from committed individuals is because prevention programs are not highly visible. Health and human service advisory boards may not be willing to give up treatment dollars for visibly ill in favor of preventive services for the general public.

However, money spent for traditional, cure-oriented alcoholic, child abuse, mental illness, emergency care, and aging programs have been no more effective than monies spent for traditional medical services. As health insurance becomes more costly and the futility of expenditures on health problems becomes obvious, the logic of prevention may become sufficiently visible.

The rising costs and health problems will only spur communities to look for alternatives. The information relating to preventive services and fitness programs and their effect on health problems must be available. The stifling of this information is still the issue and the medical profession is not alone in its influence on de-emphasizing health maintenance and disease prevention programs. The corridors of Congress are filled with lobbyists representing many business organizations and industries that prosper on the ignorance of the people.

An example is the Senate Select Committee on Nutrition Needs, chaired by Senator George McGovern. An intensive research campaign by this group led to conclusions long espoused by many health experts. They included the finding that half of all cancer cases may be related to the diet. In all, the committee found that six of the ten leading causes of death in the United States were linked to diet. Specifically, the committee recommended a decrease in the consumption of meat, whole milk, and eggs.

These dietary recommendations were submitted and shortly afterwards a hostile Congress voted the committee out of existence. The dietary recommendations themselves were subsequently changed and watered down. The recommendation to decrease the consumption of meat was removed entirely. A commitment from the head of the National Cancer Institute to inform the public about evidence that excessive calories, alcohol, and fat may increase the risk of cancer has not yet been realized.

The reason for such irresponsible reactions may have been the influence of powerful opposition from meat and dairy industries. "Economic ruination of the United States" was touted and the health of the American people was sold out for profit and political power. When the "Dietary Goals" are finally popularized by the American Health Foundation, they may not represent the totality of the original report.

This is only one example of many. Millions of Americans are misled every day by advertising that is edited by dairy and meat producers, cereal companies, grocery manufacturers, and their powerful associations. Millions of dollars are spent by these as well as by alcoholic beverage producers, tobacco companies, and fast food chains to keep people uninformed about the hazards of sugar, smoking, additives, and diet. The profit motive seems to have little regard for repercussions, whether they be a gradual decline of health or the violent reactions of a child hypersensitive to the sugars and additives promoted on Saturday morning television.

STRATEGY

Creating community awareness of legitimate health needs is a priority that must be invoked before the community can be expected to participate in exercise and health education programs.

The initial responsibility for community fitness programs must come from civic leaders and committed individuals who can inspire communicative agencies to initiate a public campaign. Existing health care agencies can be enlisted to promote health and fitness concepts that are consistent with the expert consensus. Volunteers can be used to set up booths for the purpose of educating people.

Whatever is used to increase community awareness, the following guidelines should be followed. An organized plan should assure consistent dissemination of information. The information should be consistent with that contained in the references listed in the bibliography of this book or with other information substantiated by appropriate authorities. If multiple agencies, individuals, and media sources are used, each should transmit identical, non-contradictory information.

It is also important that statements can be defended against counter-claims. Even though there may be a high correlation between heart disease and inactivity, for example, conclusive claims cannot be made. For example, it can be stated that inactivity gives rise to atrophy of certain tissues, to reduced cardiac function, and increased fatigability, but it cannot be stated that regular activity alone can prevent or cure heart disease.

It is unfortunate that such nit-picking is required. Many physicians are not so critical of "proof" in prescribing drugs that have been tested on far poorer grounds than those related to risk factors of lifestyle. However, formidable opposition demands that the game must be played. If the emphasis of the public awareness campaign is on functional capacity as opposed to disease prevention and longevity, then the messages relating to lifestyle, nutrition, and exercise are irrefutable. Functional capacity, self-esteem, and happiness, then, should be the major campaign theme. Until incontrovertible evidence is produced, this approach will prevent a loss of credibility when other announcements express doubts as to the validity of certain studies. This will prevent the confidence that may have taken months to build up from being ruined overnight.

An example of a "safe" educational package describing the benefits of exercise is published by the Swedish National Board of Health and Welfare and is entitled *Diet and Exercise*. Note the use of the word "may" and that each claim is related to clinical manifestations. The pamphlet states that regular exercise:

- counteracts obesity
- facilitates the treatment of obesity
- may prevent or reduce effects of coronary heart disease
- may reduce fatigue
- improves the peripheral circulation
- may reduce swelling of the legs
- increases the strength of involved tendons and muscle attachments
- may reduce the risk of joint injuries
- increases the muscular strength
- may give protection against back injuries and back trouble in general

Other statements might include:

- may have a positive influence on the treatment and prevention of depression
- facilitates the treatment of alcoholism and tobacco addiction
- may improve self-esteem and interpersonal relationships
- may augment learning potential in children

The public awareness strategy should attempt to use simplified slogans and poster-pictures whenever possible. Pages of information are often not read by the average citizen. For example, one poster observed in a magazine simulated a "welcome to Marlboro country" advertisement. It was identical to a typical advertisement in every way but one. All the cowboys were in beds in a coronary unit. This shows that the powerful tools of commercial advertising might be used as effectively for selling fitness as for selling products that destroy fitness.

Target populations should also be selected as they are by commercial enterprises. The major areas of concern in promoting self-responsibility for health include:

Fat control. It should be pointed out that ten billion dollars are spent annually on fraudulent "diet" products and equipment.

Self-Esteem. People care less about health than they do about self-

esteem. An awareness campaign should attempt to relate self-responsibility for health with self-esteem. For example, it can be pointed
out that there is not much honor in being taken advantage of by a
phony weight reduction scheme.

Smoking. People should realize that fitness programs, diet, and exercise can do much more to help a person quit smoking than mere
willpower. Since many people now desire to quit smoking because
they are already aware of the need in this area, an important market
exists for this approach.

Children. People should be aware of the potential harm done to
their children by smoking, sugar, and other negative addictions.
People might support a fitness program for the sake of their children
more readily than for their own sake.

Advertisement of fitness programs existing in other areas. If fitness
programs exist within business, industry, and schools, people within
the community should know about it. If the programs are successful, people within the community, but not involved, may feel as
though they are being left out of something important.. This may also
set the stage for community fitness programs.

Positive Atmosphere. People should realize that the "health care
rip-off" exists all around them, but the awareness should be promoted with a minimum of negative accusations. If people are told
that a fifteen minute walk is equal to a standard dosage of valium,
they don't need to be told that the physician who recommends
valium instead of exercise is irresponsible. If people who are eating
junk foods and not exercising are told that they are weak and ignor-
ant, it is not likely they will be responsive to the program. It is more
likely that they will retaliate.

Every attempt at promoting public awareness should appreciate
the need for positive community attitudes and support. If properly
managed, the support of the medical community can be pledged.
The awareness that physicians can do little to alleviate the major
ills of modern society does not take anything away from their
tremendous capabilities of healing. The physician is and should be a
respected member of the community, and his support can usually
be depended on if he or she is properly approached. In a community
situation it is not likely a physician will retaliate overtly. It will be
a long while before the program will take away too many of his
customers, or so he will believe.

Americans have a tremendous energy for taking a new idea and
running with it. Maximize this enthusiasm and direct it to an appreciation of self-responsibility for health and happiness.

12

COMMUNITY FOUNDATIONS

Stimulating an understanding about health care problems and solutions without an understanding of community roots, is like building a castle on a decaying foundation. Each community has its own heritage that has evolved over a long period of time. In many instances these cultural habits and attitudes contradict the goals of health and fitness and, ultimately, happiness.

Identifying patterns of behavior that are deeply rooted within the community does not require a social psychologist. It will require an individual or group familiar with the community and perceptive enough to see within the community's institutionalized foundations.

For example, a community might contain a large number of alcohol abusers. Such a population will have developed attitudes that are supportive of heavy drinking. Such attitudes may have developed a community image of the drinker that associates the drinker with masculinity, comaraderie, vitality, excitement, and sociability.

Simply making the public aware of the health hazards of alcohol and offering programs designed to cure individual drinking problems may not overcome the stronger cultural and environmental defenses. These defenses, or images, might need to be "attacked" as well. Posters and slogans can be used to identify the cultural contradictions. For example, a slogan might read, "If getting drunk is so much fun, why not start your child out on the right foot—buy him a fifth of whiskey for his or her tenth birthday."

Such a statement reveals the shallowness of the drinking image. Although the campaign should be designed to prevent the effort from becoming an enemy to the community, the truth should hurt just enough to stimulate thinking about the logic of sanctioned lifestyles. Once the contradictions surface, resistance to change will be less tenacious.

Another example of cultural attitudes that can be subversive to community fitness programs has to do with women. In many communities a woman concerned about a lack of energy or a potential cardiac risk is merely advised to "slow down" or to take tranquilizers. She is reminded that women are not susceptible to heart disease and told not to think about it. The idea of one of the community's women running around the block may be considered radical or unladylike.

Dr. Evalyn Gendel has said that the sociocultural mystique surrounding physical prowess in women is deeply embedded in our society. Although the female Olympian is now praised, the non-athlete female is still influenced by negativism and indifference. These hangovers from the past must be addressed before fitness programs are offered to women in the community.

In the attempt to change these kinds of cultural attitudes, it must be appreciated that they exist for a reason. They exist to provide an emotional crutch with which to support lifestyles that are rationally unsupportable. "Reaction formation" via the adherence to an opposite and by self-deception is a classical psychological defense mechanism for maintaining self-esteem. When attempting to remove such a crutch, care should be taken to provide an alternative support. In this case the alternative is the fitness program.

The crutch, however, must be removed. How can people learn to take responsibility for their own health if they continue to deceive themselves? Human behavior is modern man's own worst enemy. The future of Western civilization is no longer threatened by disease and famine. Instead, self-destruction looms in the form of hostility, depression, drug addiction, anxiety, hopelessness, and misdirection. Each of these ills is somehow supported by the very society that abhors them.

MENTAL WELL-BEING IN A CHANGING WORLD

These problems of living are often referred to as being symptoms of "mental" or "emotional" illness. They are not attributable to disease, but to a basic contradiction between the positive potentiality of man and his culture. A rational evaluation of this contradiction may provide the impetus for treatment and prevention of these problems through the organization of community fitness programs. Not only can such an evaluation help prepare a community for a successful fitness program, but a significant and immediate health problem can be attacked in the process. More than fifty percent of all hospital beds are filled with people diagnosed as emotionally ill. A larger percentage of illness in the home is attributable to such problems.

It has been claimed by Toffler and others that these psychological and sociological problems are a result of "future shock." This "shock" reflects the rapid accumulation of advancing technology and the resulting challenge to the moral foundations of society. Technological changes have made these foundations unstable and impermanent. Anxiety and frustration have replaced security and contentment.

Attributing the current mental health problems to rapidly increasing technology, is, however, only partially valid. It is true that the problem has increased with technological advancements. Census statistics show that twice as many Americans were treated for emotional illness in 1974 as in 1944. However, the "future shock" theory masks a more fundamental problem. It misdirects the search for the real cause by focusing attention on technological control alone.

The inherent problem has to do with the contradictory nature of the cultural foundations themselves, not the rapid influx of new information and choices resulting from technological change. The parallel increase in emotional illness and technological progress only indicates that advanced scientific information has forced people to glimpse at the contradictions and has not given them viable alternatives. The problem is that rather than challenge long standing beliefs, many individuals have chosen to escape from the momentary glance at truth. Berelson says that man distorts his understanding of the world through defense mechanisms to protect himself from what he cannot bear to face.

What is worse is that society condones this escape regardless of the consequences. In fact, many of man's institutions, his social and moral foundations, were designed for that purpose. Religion and marriage, for example, have often equated faith with knowledge. They were intended to give man structure, stability, and direction in the absence of wisdom. They were intended to confine man to a "safe" mode of behavior.

In the absence of knowledge about himself and the world, these institutions offered security. But now, technological wisdom has provided man with a byproduct of sociological wisdom. In light of this new wisdom the institutional basis for action is causing catastrophic repercussions.

But why is this basis of action a causal factor in today's mental health problem? There are two important reasons. The first has to do with man's inherent ability to reason, or to think without contradiction. To make man consciously aware of an idea that cannot be integrated into this reasoning process is, according to Branden, to "sabotage the integrative function of consciousness; to undercut one's convictions and kill one's capacity to be certain of anything." In other words, if one's faith is contradicted by those concepts of reality that have been understood through reason and experience, one becomes emotionally disturbed.

The "disturbing" factor is man's resistance to changing that in which he has an emotional stake. The resistance is especially strong when the emotional stake relates to human affairs as opposed to technological considerations. For example, Dr. Thomas Lilly was awarded prizes for his nitrogen analyzer, the Lilly Manometer (it measures changes in cabin pressure) and his device for determining the micromelting point of drugs. However, he encountered a furor for his work in interspecies communication, human emotion, and operations of the brain. It is in such areas that emotional security has its greatest stake.

Perhaps this is why, as Toynbee states, "Human affairs are still the Dark Continent of the Universe, compared to the realm of Physical nature which has been so brilliantly illuminated by the discoveries of modern science." The point is, however, that the intensity of today's scientific "illumination" is revealing the falsity of our sociological basis. Hiding in the shadows of ignorance and irrational behavior is no longer palatable to man's inherent ability to reason.

The second reason, describing why the "institutional" basis of action is a causal factor in emotional illness, is a fundamental extension of the first. It has to do with the contradiction between man's institutions and his natural behavior. The most basic wants of mankind, according to Dr. Murray Banks, include a desire to live and be healthy, a feeling of importance, a desire to be loved, and a desire for variety. In each instance, however, culture has established values that stifle these basic needs. The basic elements of good health, exercise and nutrition, have been ignored. Individual importance has been disregarded. Initiative has been stifled. People are too apprehensive of others to find love. And variety is the very antithesis of many institutions, including religion, marriage, and education.

Education is often responsible for promulgating and sanctioning the hypocrisy that nourishes mental illness. The educational process teaches an individual to function in the society as it is without ever questioning it. Information that does not fit into the established pattern is hidden. Psychology avoids philosophy.

Responsibility for such education rests with every individual and organization that teaches uninvestigated doctrines as if they were absolute truths. For example, it is the parent who causes the child to withdraw into an autistic world because he has been taught that his body is evil and asking questions is impudent. It is religious instruction that causes a woman to commit suicide because she believes the earth is a place of misery and sin. It is the public school that reinforces the competitive philosophy to "win" at all costs. It is our society that intensifies the jealousy and guilt of adultery.

Such values contradict the very nature of man. They confuse his rationality. A child is taught to avoid the evils of "self-abuse;" yet it is not the act but the teaching that will lead to behavioral problems. A man is taught to be industrious all his life; yet when he achieves a fortune he is scorned and taught that heaven has no room for the rich.

The medical profession has played a role in maintaining the status quo of irrational educative values. Preventive medicine, for example, is just beginning to be taught and practiced. Many psychologists still refuse to consider that a rational code of morality may be possible. Those who do recognize the possibility avoid the matter by claiming that man is not yet ready to take on the responsibility of a rational code of behavior. For example, Dr. William Zeller, Director of Psychology Education at the Institute of Living in Hartford, has stated:

> "Culturally and collectively we are not mature enough to discard completely old values for new. The 'wisdom of the ages' is handed down from one generation to the next, primarily to safeguard human life and give it dignity."

If man is not mature enough it is because his growth has been stifled by such educational assumptions. Such an answer is like stilling the questioning mind of a child with the reply, "It is true because I told you so" or "wait until you are older." If the current rate of emotional illness is any indication, it may be too late if man waits any longer to investigate his "old values." It may be that faith in the "wisdom of the ages" is more responsible for jeopardizing life and dignity than safeguarding it.

Thus, portions of our entire educational system, from the home to the school, either sanction contradictory values or reject ideas that might challenge existing beliefs and habits. It is these uninvestigated cultural habits that are stifling man's potentiality to accommodate more important values and more valid beliefs. Man has lost or rejected wisdom and replaced it with mythology. Father Gannon, president of Fordham University, has phrased it simply; "Culture is what is left when everything you have been taught is forgotten."

POSITIVE POTENTIALITY

If man is to replace his old values with new, the new values must have a definable basis that is both valid and non-contradictory. The phrase "positive potentiality" describes such a basis. Positive potentiality describes man's ability to achieve that which can be considered universally good. Such goals include health, love, peace, music, art, and creativity. Positive potentiality includes man's ability to discern the difference between what is good and what is not. The fact that man's irrational behavior often causes him to make the wrong decision does not preclude the existence of his ability to make the right decision. The fact that negative potentialities also exist in man is not a reason to inhibit his entire potential.

The inhibiting of positive potentiality is, in fact, an expression of negative potentiality. The English philosopher William Dunmore said that "the predicament of the whole human race is due to one shortcoming; the inability of each member of that race to express his full positive and creative mental potential."

Similarly, Dr. William S. Beck has said, "The essence of crisis is a disproportionality between the amount of misery men suffer and the potentiality of their culture." It is this potentiality that includes man's ability to reason, to achieve his basic wants, to gain knowledge and wisdom, and to realize the virtues that have been stifled by the antiquated institutions and educational philosophies of today.

It may be true that the road on which one must travel to express positive potentiality is difficult. It requires open-mindedness, courage, determination, and optimism. The road that represents an expression of negative potentiality is, unfortunately, an easier road to travel. It is easier because it is full of directional signs from our "protecting" culture. It can be traveled blindly if one has faith in the directions. The problem is that it is a dead end street.

One reason for this unfortunate irony is that things such as courage and optimism are difficult prescriptions to provide. However, there is a methodology that can inspire the realization of such concepts that may be conducive to the replacement of old values with new. For the individual this treatment means the realization of *minor success* that will directly result from a philosophy of positive potentiality.

Minor success simply refers to the accomplishment of a task that represents a partial realization of an individual's positive potential. The individual's own recognition of this accomplishment promotes self-esteem, optimism, courage, and a rational basis for faith in his own potential.

This method is as effective in preventing emotional disorders as it is in treating them. When used in child rearing it can mean the difference between a child who is able to cope and one who is not. The child is directed to attempt a task that he is physically able to perform. He is taught that accomplishment of the task is significant. Upon achievement of the task the child perceives his own ability to achieve further.

The same psychology applies to the adult. The directed accomplishments can include anything in the realm of positive potentiality, including a successful attempt at love, understanding, creativity, or the attainment of physical health. They should not include any "accomplishments" that are supportive of the contradictions that have been discussed. The concept of winning, for example, can imply both positive and negative values.

Of all the possibilities, however, the best methodology for achieving minor success involves the development of the physical health potential. There are several reasons why this approach is considered the best. The most obvious is that the attainment of physical health is easier to direct and measure than love, understanding, or creativity.

Almost any individual can be taught to improve his or her physical health. For most individuals such improvement may be extremely significant. The predominance of atherosclerosis may testify to this fact. It is also safe to assume that most individuals suffering from emotional problems are in poor physical condition.

The attainment of physical health is easy to direct and to measure. Proper exercise programs can significantly reduce resting pulse rates, blood pressure, and obesity. A simple progress chart will evidence accomplishments that are a direct result of an individual's own efforts. Properly educated as to what these minor successes indicate, the individual becomes self-motivated to continue his efforts. Realization of his own positive potentiality, and a newly acquired responsibility for one's own health, may significantly alter the course of irrational behavior.

Another reason that this physical fitness methodology may be an effective tool for restructuring values has to do with the increased opportunities for living that may not have previously been available. The individual's increased fitness may now allow him or her to participate in such activities as hiking, swimming, dancing, skiing, and others. A new appearance may instill personal confidence. The increased feeling of well-being may diminish problems that now appear significant.

Furthermore, there may even be a physiological basis for treatment and prevention of emotional disorders via a physical fitness program. Researchers have proven the relaxing effect of physical exercise. There are other chemical changes relating to exercise and diet that may significantly affect behavior. Dr. Cooper, Dr. deVreis, and Dr. Kostrubella have demonstrated a successful relationship between exercise and alcoholism, senility, and even psychosis.

The reasonably high probability regarding the effectiveness of this approach should offer a serious challenge to more traditional approaches. But psychology is still guided by assumptions that are supportive of uninvestigated cultural values. One of these values has to do with the validity of human emotions as a basis of action. The trend has been to accept human emotion as a valid basis of action. The philosophy of positive potentiality and non-contradictory behavior, however, affirms that there is only one emotion that is a valid basis for action, and that emotion relates to the concept of love.

Love is a valid basis for action because it can be considered as universally good. It is thus in the realm of man's positive potentiality. All other emotions, including anxiety, frustration, fear, hate, and jealousy are meant to serve as warning systems only. They prepare and defend man against those things that might threaten his well-being. They should stimulate the instinctive reasoning process to direct appropriate action. They should not be a basis of action per se.

Unfortunately, this theory continues to be disregarded. Man has mistakenly convinced himself that it is easier to cling to the security of his emotions than to investigate their origins. This belief is further illustrated by the many therapy groups that lure almost one million Americans each year. Underlying this entire movement is "an imperative to act spontaneously with one's feelings." Thus instead of providing the individual with the means to truly "get in touch" with oneself, the "encounter group" may do just the opposite. By putting down reason in place of emotion these groups are simply providing people with another form of irrational escape.

Similarly, the success of occult practices in this country illustrates the continuing priority of emotion over reason. But even when such practices are questioned, the basis of the doubt remains in harmony with the cultural values of uninvestigated faith. For example, Jan Ehrenwald, a psychiatrist at Roosevelt Hospital in New York, has said that the tendency for people to turn to the occult is "an expression of the chaotic state of our civilization—the loss of spititual and religious values." To the contrary; such a tendency is an extension of these spititual and religious values! Such a statement further illustrates the paradoxical avoidance of a rational basis of behavior.

Therefore, we can only avoid contradiction if we are willing to release our emotional stakes and let reason, love, and other positive potentialities guide our actions. Faith in fixed and permanent institutions that stifle such potentialities must be re-evaluated. Man is controlled by his culture only to the extent that he has set forth the conditions. There is now a need for a new set of conditions.

It is true that man must clearly define his technological goals. He must learn to control his technological capabilities. He must be aware of the potentially negative repercussions. But first he must learn to understand and control his own behavior. He must reconstruct a non-contradictory foundation on which scientific advancement and mental well-being can flourish together in harmony.

Before people will participate in community fitness programs on a large scale, they must be willing to let go of those "crutches" and emotional stakes that maintain self-esteem in spite of poor health and unhappiness. They must believe that they have the potential to be healthy and happy in spite of themselves.

13

PROGRAM IMPLEMENTATION

The point has been made that fitness programs must relate to personal experience if they are to be successful. Education alone does not necessarily lead to desirable changes of behavior. The attainment of health and fitness wisdom can occur only when knowledge is given meaning by applying it to personal experience.

As the previous chapter revealed, personal experience itself must be evaluated before such knowledge can be effectively applied. The first steps toward developing a community fitness program should include educational activities that cause people to reflect on their social values. Utmost in any approach to "values clarification" is the identification and avoidance of hypocrisy and half-truths.

This last priority is applicable not only to deep-seated attitudes and convictions but to conscious commitments to fitness improvement as well. An individual who desires to improve his or her health should be convinced that the effort will fail if half-truths and hypocrisy exist. For example, there are many people regularly shopping in "health food stores" for bushels of vitamins and special tonics who never exercise. There are people who profess to eat food that is healthy, who actually eat highly processed, additive-laden foods. There are people who do not allow their children to smoke but will surround their child with smoke from morning to night.

It is equally important that organizers of community fitness programs avoid such pitfalls. They themselves must exemplify the tenets of healthful lifestyles and exercise habits. The program will lose its credibility if its directors continue smoking and fail to exercise regularly.

Similarly, an attempt should be made to assure a congruence between the fitness message and the communications media. If magazines are to be used for health education, the reputation of the magazine and its sponsors should be considered. If an organization is solicited to give support to the program, the organization should itself be involved in promoting fitness in other ways. For example, Blue Cross and Blue Shield are involved in a major advertising campaign that stresses the importance of exercise and healthful lifestyle. They also publish recommendations for employee fitness programs. The effectiveness of this campaign, however, is nullified to a large degree when it is noted that they do not back up their health messages with premium reductions for fit individuals and that they do not themselves have an employee fitness program.

Words and actions should be compatible. Once fitness education is recognized as a sincere, consistent message from reliable, non-contradictory sources, a greater tendency toward its acceptance will occur. People must have faith in a system if they are going to turn their lives over to it.

PHYSICAL FITNESS COMMITTEE

Just as developing a fitness committee is an appropriate first step in organizing fitness programs in business, so it is in developing programs for communities. The committee can be started by any interested citizen willing to commit some time and energy to improving the well-being of a community. Members can be solicited from the community at large or from existing health care organizations.

The prospect of selecting members from the community at large may have several advantages over using individuals from other health care organizations. The primary advantage is that members not previously affiliated with another health agency are less apt to have political or biased motives. Secondly, individuals who have served on various city or county health care boards and committees may have preconceptions about the potential influence of a single committee.

A newspaper ad requesting volunteers to work on a committee that will attempt to design a fitness program for the community may have a surprisingly large response. There may be many people within the community who would appreciate the opportunity to play a part in this project. There might even be individuals serving on existing councils who, frustrated by a lack of progress with their own traditional program, would resign to join the new committee. For example, in Marin County, California, each of the health and human services committees has given lip service to prevention through health education and fitness programs. None have taken action in these areas and the few supporters of such programs remain frustrated. Perhaps a committee especially designed toward this end would provide the answer to this frustration.

In addition to general membership, an attempt should be made to solicit key figures from community government and from local medical facilities. This will serve the political interests of the committee during its attempt to elicit funds and may also provide some helpful direction.

Once the committee has been formed, it should then be formally recognized by local government and by various health and educational agencies. In gaining this recognition it is important for the committee to announce a plan that will emphasize cooperation, not competition with the various agencies. In this way a maximum amount of support might be expected and a minimum amount of political resistance. There is no doubt that exercise, nutrition, and lifestyle education is fundamentally involved with such community programs as the Committee on Aging, Drug Abuse, Alcohol Abuse, Child Abuse, Emergency Medical Care, Heart Associations, Cancer Society Committees, Mental Illness, etc. Although these committees are usually caught up in their own traditional treatment modalities, each would be supportive of the fitness committee in some degree, and mutual energy might be productive for all concerned.

HEALTH SYSTEMS AGENCY

The physical fitness committee should also ally itself with the local health systems agency. In most instances the committee would be welcomed as an official sub-committee to the agency. The provisions of the law that established the HSAs distinctly legitimize their involvement in activities that relate to exercise, nutrition, and lifestyle education and promotion.

There are several advantages related to an association with an HSA. Funding may occasionally be acquired for specific operations proposed by a fully designated HSA. An HSA sub-committee will be in a better position to receive monies than an outside committee. Although competition for the money will be high, even within the agency, a strong committee leadership might be able to obtain funding for one of several fitness projects.

A second advantage is the availability of a paid staff for helping with printed materials, mailings, and research. The use of these tools can be of great help to a committee that is operating without any funding.

The third advantage of HSA affiliation has to do with committee members' participation on Certificate of Need Review Panels. Certificates of Need, according to the law, will be required by any hospital or public health agency that wishes to make a significant financial expenditure. The proposal must go before a designated panel that will make recommendations to the state as to the merit of the proposal. Herein lies what little power the HSAs have.

Unfortunately, this power of restraint rings a negative chord among health care professionals. Also, there is always a law and a lawyer who can overcome restraints of this nature. However, it would be easier for a health care facility to comply with stipulated agency priorities in many cases than to invoke legal complications. This would be especially true if the priorities implemented by the review panel emphasized health maintenance and education. Such programs would be relatively easy to facilitate and would have little public opposition.

For example, a community hospital might want to add a coronary unit. The established need for an additional coronary unit in the community may be marginal. Although the hospital desires the extra income and growth potential, the panel may decide that there is already a sufficient number of coronary units. The hospital may be on unsteady grounds.

If, however, the hospital can build into the proposal something that meets the high priorities of the Certificate of Need panel, the chances for approval may be better. Using the health education priority, the hospital could, with a nominal budget increase, provide a significant health education program for heart disease prevention to augment the coronary care unit. A comprehensive program might include out-patient education in waiting rooms and during office consultations. It might include specific exercise, nutrition, and lifestyle information regularly provided to coronary patients.

If the physical fitness committee could influence the panel, or participate on the panel in such a way as to give the panel the reputation for adhering to the health maintenance priority in its decisions, every petitioner might seriously begin to modify its proposals to include some measure for health education and fitness promotion. In this way the negative power of HSAs could be turned into a positive power. Incentives, not regulations, would provide impetus.

There is also a disadvantage to working under the auspices of one of the health systems agencies. In most instances the agencies spend more time interpreting state and federal regulations and developing by-laws in accordance with these regulations than they do imple-
committee can avoid such pitfalls, it might be more productive for

it to remain independent. A strong committee can still gain financial support from local government and from private and public funding institutions.

FUNDING ALTERNATIVES

Depending upon the size of the community and the degree of voluntary service, the fitness committee will probably need to consider various kinds of financial support. Generally speaking, funding alternatives can be categorized as follows:

1. Federal Funding;
- Public Health Service Act
- Consumer Health Education and Information Act
- Economic Opportunity Act
- Community Mental Health Center Act
- Special Grants
   2. Foundation Grants
   3. Special Tax Fund
   4. Y.M.C.A.
   5. Community Sponsored
   6. Private Enterprise

Another federal funding possibility is under the auspices of the Economic Opportunity Act of 1964. Under this act the creation of "neighborhood health centers" was intended to provide an innovative use of community participation in policy making and staffing for individual and community health care. The center hires family health workers who promote health education, patient care, and social advocacy activities in individual homes. Although the community health centers typically practice only traditional medicine, their intent would by definition have to support a health maintenance and physical fitness concept.

The concept of a community health center has also been developed within the field of mental health. Centers funded under the Community Mental Health Centers Act of 1963 provide such programs as family-crisis intervention, suicide prevention, and psychological counseling to a fourth of the population. The goals of the act include providing a range of coordinated preventive and rehabilitative services. Considering the increased awareness and knowledge relating mental health to physical fitness, the community mental health centers should begin to initiate this type of treatment and prevention modality. In addition to this incentive the Kennedy ammendment to Title XVI of the Public Health Service Act notes that there has been a "lack of coordination" between mental and physical health planning and suggests an appropriate modification in future mental health care.

The major responsibility for initiating a community mental health center rests with the local community. Citizens, agencies, or organizations interested in developing a center should contact both the regional office of the United States Department of Health, Education and Welfare, which provides consultation and assistance in making an application to the National Institute of Mental Health for a construction grant, and the state agency that has drawn up a statewide plan for center construction, which provides information regarding the priority of the local community for construction funds in the state plan based on the need for services and on the adequacy of existing facilities. In the case of a staffing grant, community members follow a similar procedure. The state mental health authority, however, only evaluates the staffing grant application and does not control the grant's funding priority.

Once a grant has been made and a center established, community members continue to play active roles in the operation of the center. They serve on advisory boards and they work as volunteers within the center. The use of community volunteers is an important element in determining the success of the program. As with most grants, some form of non-federal maintenance funding should be developed. For example, charging small sums for ongoing fitness assessment could be considered once the value of such evaluations has been established within the community.

The concept of community health action programs is growing in importance as more experiments are proving themselves worthy. If the programs are too successful on a large scale, however, they will need to expand the horizons of traditional health care to include physical fitness programs. Until all national and local health care programs accept the broadened definition of health that includes physical, social, and psychological well-being, they are all doomed to failure and a waste of money.

In addition to federal grants there are many foundation grants periodically available throughout the country. Most of the grants are applicable to improving the holistic well-being of people and most would consider a proper proposal to implement a community fitness program. The Rockefeller Foundation, for example, is very interested in community health center concepts. Information about such grants can be obtained from local health agencies, universities, and human services organizations.

For those who have an aversion to governmental affiliation, or where federal funds are not available through grants, there are still several possibilities for program development and implementation. Of these a local Y.M.C.A. offers the most credible, prestructured vehicle for providing a community with a comprehensive fitness program.

Although many local Y.M.C.A.s have not yet implemented it, the National Board of the Y.M.C.A. has developed the best program for improving the health and fitness of Americans. The Nationwide Y.M.C.A. Cardiovascular Health Program was developed by some of the top health and fitness experts in the world. The program includes five major segments:

- "Y.M.C.A. Feelin' Good Program" for youth.(see part 6).
- "Y.M.C.A. Activities," which focuses on weight reduction through physical activity.
- "The Y's Way to Physical Fitness" which is a program of standardized fitness testing and exercise activities.

The goal of the Y.M.C.A. is to have more than eight million persons actively engaged in specific health enhancement programs by 1980. If this goal is to be reached, Y.M.C.A.s will need the support of communities and organizations like a physical fitness committee.

There are often other agencies in addition to the Y.M.C.A. that could be used as a base of operations for developing a community fitness program. If enough volunteer personnel could be involved in promoting a fitness program, the community itself, through donations, bond issues, or local government funding could afford staff, materials, and space sufficient for starting a program.

If a community cannot be stimulated into publicly supporting a fitness program, and if grant funding is not available, the physical fitness committee might consider a private enterprise using a strict fee-for-service approach. Legitimate adult fitness programs have a great potential for profit within a community as well as for offering a worthwhile service.

Beginning a fitness business requires basically the same personnel, equipment, and facilities as have been described previously. If quality assessment and exercise prescription are offered in combination with meaningful education and enthusiastic, charismatic leadership, people will partake of the service. In some instances, a business could be developed to franchise a testing and educational package to various health spas within a community that, like most commer-

cial health spas, are not offering such quality education and motivation.

COMMUNITY COOPERATION

Regardless of the source of funding or the nature of the base of
operations, a successful community fitness program must be at
least visible to the majority of the population. All of the health and
human service agencies within the community should endorse the
fitness program as an important and legitimate health care alternative. Every attempt should be made to involve all of the existing
recreation clubs and sports organizations. The program should not
be a competitive threat to existing gymnasiums and health spas but
should augment their facilities. A fitness program is basically educational. People will still want attractive, diversified exercise alternatives.

Community hospitals should be approached by the committee
and requested to assist with implementing health education in its
own policies. In many instances hospitals have a "captive audience"
and the use of health educators, health psychologists, physicians,
and nurses to provide the patient with information relating to
disease prevention would have significant impact. A policy should be
evoked where the traditional passive patient can be stimulated to
take a more active role in his or her health.

Hospitals should also be encouraged to provide services and facilities consistent with the community health program. The Senate
Committee on Nutrition and Human Needs found that malnutrition
in hospitals demonstrates "stark evidence" of medical neglect of
nutrition. The American Health Foundation reported that not a
single hospital in New York City offered a smoking cessation program. In many hospitals smoking is permitted, even in rooms where
there are patients suffering from diseases caused or aggravated by
smoking.

Similarly, many hospitals provide vending machines that sell
cigarettes and "junk food." How could a diabetic being admitted
to such a hospital ever be expected to believe that there is any other
remedy for diabetes other than medical treatment? A Rockefeller
Foundation report claimed that a hospital patient education program
for diabetics could reduce readmission rates by fifty percent. How
could a successful education program exist with such hypocrisies
in evidence?

The fitness committee should be sure to include hospitals in its
list of fitness promotion targets for community involvement. As Mr.
Carlson states in *The End of Medicine,* "There is no opportunity for
recreation or exercise in a hospital and there is little opportunity to

be outdoors...The modern hospital is one of the unhealthiest places around."

The communications media should also be used to great advantage. Community service space in papers and magazines as well as time on radio and television can be used to promote the fitness program. Slogans and educational reminders should barrage the community until everyone knows about the program and its benefits.

The actual exercise program can become a community project. Neighborhoods and police departments can facilitate weekend bicycle rides over traffic controlled streets. Running clubs can sponsor fun runs for people of all abilities. Discounts to spas, sports clubs, and events can be given to fitness program participants. Colleges and universities can offer their facilities for public use at convenient times. Housewives can take turns babysitting while other mothers take regular walks or runs and bicycle rides. Restaurants could be requested to publish the nutritional and caloric content of their menus. The alternatives for promoting and assisting the fitness program are limited only by imagination and concern.

That such programs can work within a community has been demonstrated. Projects like that conducted by Stanford's Dr. Farquar in the community of Watsonville, California have proven that entire communities can significantly reduce risk factors such as inactivity, smoking, stress, and poor diet with community involvement and media support. Unfortunately, such projects have received little acclaim and little cash. They require the dedication, concern, and participation of large numbers of individuals within the community. Bypass valve operations may get the glory and the money, but community fitness programs can bring the health and happiness.

UNDERLYING PRINCIPLES

If certain basic, underlying principles are fully understood by all people directly involved in developing and implementing a community fitness program, then the ultimate success of the program is all but guaranteed. Even a properly managed program with proper testing protocols and educational programs could fail if these principles are not understood. Overzealousness, a failure to appreciate environmental considerations, and a narrow focus on the role of fitness could each bring doom to an otherwise ideal program. These basic principles are well worth discussing further.

1. Well-being must not be considered an anti-doctor or antimedicine strategy. According to Ardell, "It seeks to define the limitations of medicine realistically, and to relieve the illness sector from

the destructive burdens of unfair expectations." In many cases leaders of the movement will be physicians themselves. Of course, there is a need for new curriculum in medical schools. At present most physicians are trained in hospitals and training a physician in a hospital is like training the forester in the lumber yard.

2. Intervening into the health of individuals involves a variety of components that must be considered. People in general, patients, physicians, insurance companies, schools, health planners and educators, health committees, and the political process all affect the health behavior of people within a community.

3. The existence of so many variables often makes an effort to change priorities in health care a difficult task. Therefore, if priorities can't be changed immediately, show how exercise and health education can affect existing priorities. For example, a Chevrolet commercial does not really sell the product but instead sells the image of "feeling good." Self-esteem is a legitimate priority. Income is a legitimate priority. These and other existing priorities should be related to the fitness program.

4. Physical fitness is not an elitist concept. The basic principles of health education, lifestyle, and exercise are as applicable to the disadvantaged as they are to the advantaged.

5. There is no easy way to optimal health. Any program that makes such a claim is probably fraudulent. Optimal health involves many factors including proper physical activity, nutrition, environment, the ability to cope with stress, levels of stress, social and psychological considerations, individual goals and assumptions, an understanding of when to use the medical system, and more.

6. The counsel of an individual or organization that is not supportive of health should not be considered either effective or valid. Somewhere in the process of implementing such counsel, a contradiction will betray the objective.

7. The climate for developing fitness programs is ideal. The financial costs of traditional health care and the increasing awareness of Americans of the benefits of exercise are all supportive.

8. Incentives, not regulations, will provide the best results. Social intervention often fails because it ignores the role of properly structured economic incentives for achieving goals. Innovative concepts providing economic incentives for being healthy must begin to replace incentives for being sick. Today, the healthy pay for the sick. The sicker someone is, the more they profit from health plans. Sick leave rewards the ill and deprives those who keep themselves healthy. Today's incentives assume a weak, passive population.

Tomorrow's incentives should assume a population that is ready to take care of itself.

9. Physical fitness programs that emphasize exercise, nutrition, and healthy habits should be considered as prevention and treatment modalities for a wide variety of health problems including emotional illness, child abuse, drug abuse, physical health, social well-being and even financial well-being. In each case an argument for involvement in a physical fitness program can be supported.

10. Health and fitness should be considered in terms of human potentiality and quality of life, not so much in terms of disease prevention and longevity in years. Health is much more than the absence of illness. It is a dynamic state of being that allows a person to do his or her best with the available capacities and to continue to try and maximize these capacities. Being in good health means to have the ability to live one's life to the fullest, to cope with reality, its pains and its pleasures, and to cherish survival without being afraid to risk it.

In terms of this last principle, the measurable benefits of a physical fitness program may be difficult to quantify. Subjective surveys relating to happiness and well-being, long-term reductions in suicide, and other possible results could never be scientifically associated exclusively with any one parameter. However, such associations can be logically significant within a community and if properly recorded could help motivate other communities to take action as well.

A primary function of the California Health Foundation is the establishment of a Community Health Index (CHI) for assessing the actual quality of life in a community. Comprised of such standards as housing conditions, state of the environment, employment trends (including frequency of job changes), income and education levels, criminal activity, civic involvement, degree of substance abuse (drugs and alcohol), and transportation systems, the CHI will serve as the human equivalent to the nation's GNP. Every business uses quantifiable standards for analyzing profit, investment return, reward to employees and stockholders, and the quality and production costs of its products or services. Just as our GNP is used in determining economic policy, the results of the CHI audit can be used by decision makers in the areas of health, human development, and environmental policymaking. As an example, there can be no remedy for infant mortality in a given community unless there is a clear focus on specific sub-areas where the incidence is greater. A comprehensive social-environmental-health audit such as the CHI could pinpoint areas where the quality of life is determined to be low, and provide the type of information necessary to raise this standard to a respectable level.

According to Dr. Andrew Mecca, director of the California Health Foundation and designer of the CHI, once a community health index is developed and tested, it can be used by each community or state, and ultimately aggregated for a National Health Index. Initially, the foundation for this vital source of information should generate from a private, and therefore objective, organization with no immediate stake in creating statistics favorable to public agencies or special interest groups.

Whatever the source, a good health index may help clarify the positive and negative influences on the quality of life. In comparison with the long-term effect of physical fitness programs, it could provide an incentive for all Americans to support and participate in physical fitness activities.

PART FOUR:

FITNESS AND AGING

14

FITNESS PROGRAMS
FOR SENIORS

There is a large and rapidly growing body of literature giving evidence for the potential contributions of physical exercise to the health of older people. Even a cursory review of that literature reveals that the physiological changes which seem to accompany the aging process and which collectively result in gross losses of functional capacity may, in many instances, be more closely associated with inactivity than to age in years.

For example, as the average person grows older, skeletal muscles decrease gradually in strength and endurance. Active muscle tissue is reduced. (In spite of this people usually allow themselves to gain weight as they grow older. With a decrease in active muscle tissue they would get fatter even if they stayed the same weight.) Most importantly, the capacity for oxygen consumption (aerobic capacity) decreases significantly. By age seventy-five men and women often lose about fifty percent of their maximal oxygen consumption.

Interestingly, many of these changes, particularly the loss of aerobic capacity, can be brought about in young, well-conditioned people by forced bed rest—in as little as three weeks. Dr. Samuel Fox, of the Cardiology Exercise Laboratory at Georgetown University, reported that one of the better studies in this area found that in three weeks of bed rest, the maximal cardiac output decreased by twenty-six percent; the maximal stroke volume of the heart during exercise by thirty percent; oxygen consumption by thirty percent; and even the amount of active tissue declined by 1.5 percent.

Thus it can be seen that inactivity can produce losses in function entirely similar to those brought about more slowly in the average individual when he or she grows more sedentary with age. These observations challenge the idea that losses in function are necessarily age changes alone and not conditions brought about by the long-term deconditioning of the increasingly sedentary life most people lead as they grow older.

According to Dr. Lawrence E. Lamb, if true aging processes and deterioration by unrecognized disease were not accompanied by dis-use, at age seventy a person may have reached only the halfway mark of the possible life span. Many disabilities of the seventy year old person are from acquired defects that are not necessarily time-dependent. The first step in managing these problems is to recognize that they are illnesses, not just the ravages of time.

The possibility of a life span capacity far in excess of what is typically seen today is further confirmed by the fact that some people do live more than a century. Many biblical characters were reported to have lived to more than one hundred fifty years of age. The Russians claim certain populations with an average life span of more than one hundred twenty-five years. A Dane, Christen Jacobsen Bragenberg, lived until the age of one hundred forty-six.

From such examples, it can be concluded that man has the biological capacity of living at least this long. Furthermore, there are many individuals more than seventy-five years of age who are still unusually vigorous, both mentally and physically. Entire populations in Ecuado, Hunza, and the Caucasus over the age of seventy-five engage in many hours of vigorous physical exertion daily. There are also many examples in the United States of people who cross-country snow ski in their nineties, climb mountains in their eighties, and run marathons in their seventies. Herman Smith, for example, also called Jack Rabbit Yohannsen, is an active cross-country skier at age one hundred three. Jack LaLanne, at age sixty-five, is performing physical feats that most young athletes cannot perform. The well-known ultramarathoner, Walt Stack, is running one hundred mile races at age seventy-two. Senior Olympic competition is seeing records being set that average teenagers cannot break.

These examples cannot be dismissed as simply resulting from heredity. According to Dr. Theodore Klumpp, heredity in this respect does nothing more than repeat internal physical or chemical patterns of action or reaction, or living habits that are conducive to longevity. In studies conducted on such individuals, genetic similarities were not among the major characteristics found to be in common among individuals having such vitality this late in life. Instead, the long-lived people who are able to indulge in regular vigorous activities and display an unusual degree of health and vitality had the following characteristics in common:

1. They engaged in many hours of vigorous physical exertion daily.

2. They were generally slender and well muscled.

3. Diets were in general much lower in fats, salt, and refined foods than the usual American diet.

Exercise may be the closest thing to an anti-aging drug in existence. Physical activity and the resultant increase in muscle mass can maintain the generation of hormones from the adrenal and sex glands. Maintaining the musculature along the spine, shoulders, and abdomen can prevent the sagging posture often associated with older people. Maintaining the optimal range of capacity of the hips and knees can prevent the loss in height associated with increasing years. Regular stretching of a joint also helps retain normal tendon length.

Physical activity also maintains the strength and function of the skeletal system. Bones that are not involved in regular physical activity tend to decalcify. If a leg is put in a cast it loses calcium. If such activity is maintained, the bone marrow will continue to form enough red blood cells each day to replace those that are destroyed.

Patterns of movement are also integrated with the nervous system. Functions of the musculoskeletal system affect the memory organization and fundamental patterns of response. Senility in those older persons described above is entirely absent. The decreased oxygen transport capabilities resulting from inactivity is also responsible for the mental impairment often associated with older individuals.

It must be noted that although hard scientific data does not explain exactly why, heart disease is virtually absent in those populations whose lifestyles incorporate high degrees of physical activity and diets restricted in fats and highly refined foods.

Whatever other factors may influence this fact, the consensus of medical research indicates that proper physical exercise increases the circulation to the heart muscle, increases the volume capacity of the heart, and enhances many other complex mechanisms that improve oxygen transport. To the extent that exercise decreases obesity and lowers the amount of fat particles in the blood, it helps to prevent the build-up of atherosclerotic plaque which causes blockage of the arteries. Proper exercise can also reduce blood pressure and help maintain the lung capacity.

THE HAPPINESS RATIONALE

In addition to the physiological benefits of a fitness program for seniors, there are psychological and sociological benefits as well. In combination with improved physical health, these benefits can mean many pleasurable and meaningful years for an individual who otherwise is often resigned to isolation, illness, and a loss of love and meaning. In his testimony before the Subcommittee on Aging, Dr. Frederick Swartz concluded his recommendations for exercise programs for older persons with the following personal comments:

"Mr. Chairman, this concludes my statement. I would like to add one sentence that may add a degree of credibility to what I have just said; because this (exercise) has been my lifestyle since World War II, I am on the job twelve or fourteen hours, seven days a week, and I just passed my seventy-third birthday."

Such a statement should be encouraging to senior citizens who have been pushed out of the mainstream of living and social functioning. Impaired mobility in middle-aged and older people resulting from relative inactivity and poor lifestyle habits leads to social isolation, personality and emotional deterioration, and poor mental health. Muscular degeneration and distortion of the body image lead to an increasing fear of any physical activity or pleasurable motor activity. This inactivity increases internal tensions and pent-up aggressions so commonly associated with older, inactive persons.

Physical activity opens up new interests, goals, skills, experiences, and abilities. It increases the independence of older persons. Performed in groups it also permits new interpersonal relationships. This increased independence and ability to relate to others without being dependent upon them provides a strong basis for good mental health.

Americans are often criticized for the apparent disrespect for their elders as exemplified by the many older individuals who are cast aside into nursing and rest homes. One out of twelve people beyond the age of sixty-five in the United States is in a nursing home, as compared to only six out of one thousand in Europe! The criticism, however, would be more appropriately aimed at the cause of the American reluctance to continue a non-institutional association with their elders.

It might be understood, for example, that a younger individual would not want to spend a significant portion of his or her life attending to the needs of a feeble and senile invalid who may need to be fed, dressed, and taken to the toilet. Indeed, this is the condition of many Americans past the age of sixty-five. If, however, an individual's elders were physically and mentally alert, as are many older Europeans, the prospect of sharing life with someone near and dear is more than wonderful. Although old age can sometimes merely make a habit out of ignorance, it can also bring forth wisdom. Many of the greatest achievements of humanity are the result of people in their seventh, eighth, and ninth decades of life.

ECONOMIC RATIONALE

Although the financial incentive for implementing fitness programs for senior citizens may be of less importance than the other reasons, it is a consideration that demands attention. Medical care resources are disproportionately allocated to those over sixty-five. In fiscal 1970, the average annual medical bill for an aged person was seven hundred ninety-one dollars, compared to one hundred twenty-three dollars for a child and two hundred ninety-six for those between nineteen and sixty-five. Sixty percent of this expenditure was from public funds. The aged account for about ten percent of the population, and receive about thirty percent of medical care expenditures. (See United States Compendium of National Health Expenditures Data).

The tragedy of this economic aspect is not in the cost alone but in the comparative misdirection of monies spent. Health care expenditures for the aged do not prevent contagious disease from spreading and do not restore functional capacity or well-being in most cases. Seven percent of the entire national health care expenditure goes to nursing homes. Other monies for the elderly go to drugs for reducing pain and postponing death only to prolong agony. Many funds are used to provide aids for mobility and manipulation, which in itself is often a tragic irony.

For example, "meals-on-wheels" is one approach chosen by Extended Services for the Elderly in Seattle. The organization, initially subsidized by the Office of Economic Opportunity, delivers meals to elderly so they do not have to do the work themselves. This type of service, and many other technological devices also used to "make life easier" for the older person, are sometimes the very causes of the person's problem. Dr. Frederick Swartz commented on this before the Subcommittee on Aging, when he claimed that one of his patients developed painful and debilitating swollen ankles after receiving "meals-on-wheels" because she stopped doing any activity.

By the year 2000 there will probably be relatively more older Americans than there are now. As medical costs continue to skyrocket, the costs of such medical support for the aged may become intolerable to the American public. Considering the care and regard for old people in this country today, there is no telling what attitudes might prevail as the situation worsens. There can be no doubt that health care policies for the elderly must begin to focus on physical activity and nutrition instead of inactivity and drugs.

THE TRAINABILITY OF OLDER PERSONS

A neighborhood project in Santa Cruz, California once involved the services of a group of children who exercised pets whose owners were unable to do it themselves. After several months, several veterinarians and pet owners claimed that the health and vitality of many older dogs who had become fat or ill with inactivity was restored. Although the moral of this story does not necessarily disprove the adage that "you can't teach an old dog new tricks," it does show that they can regain those abilities they once had.

Notwithstanding the point that is made, an analogy between the learning capability of man and dog is inappropriate. Many older individuals have taken up dancing, hiking, cross-country skiing, swimming, horseback riding, and other activities for the first time in their lives. Tolstoy began riding a bicycle at age sixty-seven. Genovita Guttieriez of San Marcos, Texas started swimming lessons at age one hundred seventeen. In any event, there is significant evidence that even for those older people who have been sedentary most of their lives, fitness can be improved by roughly the same percentages as is usually observed in the young.

TRAINABILITY OF INDIVIDUALS
WITH DIAGNOSED HEART DISEASE

It is estimated that twenty-seven million Americans, or one-eighth of the population, suffer from some form of cardiovascular disease. Most of these cases have not been diagnosed. If everyone with heart disease, whether diagnosed or not, were advised not to properly exercise, the tragic waste of human potential would continue or worsen. With all the conflicts of opinion about heart disease and the medical warnings against unsupervised exertion, however, many individuals are, in fact, afraid to engage in physical activity.

Aside from the fact that the majority of heart attacks occur during sleep, post-coronary exercise therapy has proven itself in large measures. Heart clinics in San Francisco and Honolulu have increased the functional capacity of literally thousands of individuals who had previously suffered a heart attack. Many individuals who could not walk from one end of a room to another without experiencing angina are now running twenty-six mile races. At the Longevity Institute in Santa Barbara, California, nutrition and exercise programs for patients are precluding the need for bypass surgery.

There are legitimate precautions that an individual with known heart disease or with multiple risk factors for coronary heart disease must take before and during participation in exercise programs. These concerns, however, focus on an understanding of proper exercise, not on the question of whether or not to exercise.

Exercise Prescription for:

_____

Name

Classification (Circle appropriate findings and recommendations):
  A. **Unrestricted exercise.** All ratings good or excellent. Well within limits in all tests. Unsupervised exercise or recreational sports activities including very heavy and extreme effort.
  B. **Fitness program.** No poor ratings. Within limits in all tests. Supervised group exercise for progressive conditioning. Calisthenics and jogging controlled by heart rate. Moderate to heavy effort.
  C. **Preconditioning program.** Poor rating in any test. Near limit in any test. Age over 60. Minor orthopedic or other problem. Individualized programs for progressive preconditioning. Walking, light jogging, swimming or bicycle ergometer exercise controlled by heart rate. Very light to light effort.
  D. **Medical review.** Poor or unusual responses to step test. Beyond limit in any test. Major orthopedic or other problem. No increased exercise or effort without physician's recommendations.

Recommended exercise _____ Heart rate _____
Duration of exercise _____
Frequency per week _____

Additional comments: _____

Agreed upon goals _____

Examiner _____
Date _____

15

DUTY CALLS

The responsibility for developing physical fitness programs for senior Americans should be assumed by various groups within the United States. These areas of responsibility include:

- federal, state, and local government
- the public health education system
- physicians and hospitals
- concerned citizens within a community
- families of older persons
- older persons themselves

Given the fact that the United States already spends more welfare dollars per person than socialized Great Britain, it is appropriate to expect that the government should contribute significantly.

There is no doubt that government could help provide for the vital need for trained exercise leaders with an understanding of the older citizen. Government funds should be available to train physical educators and other professionals concerned with exercise in aging Americans. There is also a need for the accumulation of scientific data from physical exercise programs to determine the best ways to intervene into the inactive lifestyle of such people.

Rather than encourage senior citizens to be active and productive in later years, society and governmental policies have pushed older Americans into a "take it easy" lifestyle that inevitably leads to a hospital, a convalescent home, or an untimely death. These Americans pay the price with their lives and society pays in hundreds of millions of dollars for medical and ancillary services that do little for productivity or happiness.

Such policies mean that the elderly do not have entirely a free choice as to whether they will remain vigorously active or not. Besides the barriers of ignorance and a lack of motivation, there are other barriers to overcome over which individuals have no control. Lack of funds, an inhospitable environment, lack of facilities, inadequate transportation, and a lack of trained supervision and leadership are some of these.

The federal government and, in some cases, state and local government, could address these needs with grants to localities, states, and other public and private agencies who would agree to plan, staff, and maintain such programs and facilities. Within a relatively few years, such grants would more than pay for themselves by reducing the heavy expenditures for medical and paramedical services for which the government is now liable. The medical evidence for this claim has already been accumulated. Failure of the government to act will only result in the costs of care for the elderly to continue to escalate.

There is already authority for the Department of Health Education and Welfare to encourage or establish programs of physical activity for the elderly. The National Health Planning Act and the Health Education Act have provisions that could be used to elicit funding for fitness programs for the elderly. Some emphasis to this concern has been legislated through the Older Americans Act of 1965 and the President's Council on Physical Fitness and Sports.

Title III of the Older Americans Act is a Federal-State formula grant program, which has as its overall objective the development or strengthening, at the sub-state level, of coordinated, comprehensive service programs for older persons. A wide range of services is identified in the law which may be provided or coordinated under this program, including the following:

- health related services
- preventive services
- recreational services
- any other services determined to be necessary for the general welfare of older persons

Physical fitness programs can be supported under Title III of the Older Americans Act, but state and local agencies on aging must determine if such activities fall within the priorities established by the needs surveys that are required as part of the state and area plan. The difficulty in changing the current priorities in these agencies has been addressed previously and should be appreciated once again in this area. However, remember that the concept of fitness programs as a viable solution to the many needs of older Americans is supportable and can be sold.

For example, West Virginia initiated a physical fitness project for the elderly under Title III in Charleston in 1970, and the project was so successful that the program (which is now supported through a variety of sources), operated by the Laurence Frankel Foundation, has expanded until it is now offered statewide, in Senior Centers, nursing homes, and state hospitals.

The President's Council on Physical Fitness and Sports is charged with the promotion and improvement of the physical fitness of all Americans. The Council has already initiated efforts toward promoting physical fitness programs for older Americans. They have sponsored Lowell Thomas radio ads promoting exercise for senior citizens. They have produced a film available for free loan entitled, "Physical Fitness for Older Americans." They have prepared a booklet, *The Fitness Challenge...in the Later Years* in conjunction with the Administration on Aging. And they have sponsored workshops throughout the United States for leadership training for physical fitness for the aging.

Government has thus acknowledged its responsibility for creating fitness programs for older Americans. It has also acknowledged a responsibility for helping to lessen the cost of medical care and other social services that have been determined ineffective and wasteful. In neither case has there been any significant gain. Every effort, however, should continue to be made to enlist governmental action that may give financial or regulatory assistance to the implementation of physical fitness programs for senior people.

PUBLIC HEALTH EDUCATION

The difference between health education and health information has been alluded to several times throughout this text. Health information is simply facts. Health education is the application of these facts to practical experience. Health education motivates a person to take the information and do something with it.

Health information applicable to older persons has grown tremendously in volume, especially as it relates to exercise. Health education has grown much more slowly. For older persons, especially those suffering from chronic ailments, the need is critical for a nationwide effort to change personal attitudes toward health and activity and to influence them to take more individual responsibility for the health of their minds and bodies by making changes in their lifestyles. The vital role physical activity can play has rarely been clearly explained or adequately dramatized.

Vehicles for educating older people about exercise are many. Retired people are often a captive audience. Educational opportunities exist wherever they congregate; in churches, at social functions, during workshops, and at various institutions. Retirement homes offer an excellent opportunity for fitness programs and education. They are already designed to provide social and recreational activities which would complement programs involving more dynamic life sustaining activities. Even the most progressive, luxurious retirement villages in the country are sorely lacking in qualified personnel and programs for enhancing physical fitness.

More and more older people are taking adult education classes that are being offered in community colleges. Here would be an excellent means of providing fitness education. Radio and television also offer an opportunity for such education. Public television programs like Hugh Downs' "Over Easy" are already aimed at the older population. All they would need is a regular segment of the program designed as an ongoing fitness and nutrition course.

A community hospital is also an excellent medium for public health education for senior citizens. Given the proper space, equipment, and personnel, the hospital could provide public lectures or courses on how to use the community's various exercise alternatives, accident prevention, nutritional guidance, and exercise testing. Selected patients could be recommended by physicians and social workers to take part in classes in fat reduction, management of diabetes, emotional problems, and other concerns that should be relegated to the fitness solution.

Of course, a prerequisite to educating hospital patients about fitness would be the education of hospital staff. The expansion of such an educational effort would be a natural evolution in hospital care. In many cases the frustration felt by nurses in dealing with older patients for whom there is typically no hope for a return to a normal living capacity could be changed into a rewarding feeling about the prospects of older patients subjected to fitness education.

PHYSICIAN RESPONSIBILITY

Private physicians control more than eighty percent of all medical services in the United States, from nursing homes to drug prescriptions. Nowhere is the current potential for educating senior citizens about nutrition and exercise greater. The "gospel" of a physician's recommendations is still highly revered by most older people who do not realize the nature of traditional medical education. If a physician were willing and able to educate his or her patients about exercise and nutrition, or at least recommend another alternative for such education, there would be many more older people enjoying a healthy existence. Physicians, and to a lesser extent other health care professions, have largely promulgated the "medical mystique." By keeping health and disease prevention and treatment a mystery to the public, they have maintained job security and an exaggerated sense of importance. The health professions would perform an extremely valuable service if they would actively disperse the aura of mystery that envelops medicine. A mere expansion of five or ten minutes an office visit would often be enough time to inform people about the limitations and effectiveness of medical and lifestyle interventions.

Although physicians must further educate themselves about nutrition and exercise, most already understand the basic relevance of various influences from exercise to drugs on the health of people. For example, a study published in the *New England Journal of Medicine* by Dr. Lewis Thomas analyzed the way medical care is used for the treatment of an internist's own family. Despite the fact that the families had ideal access to the medical system and had basically the same incidence of illness, most did not have regular routine physical examinations, few had been X-rayed (except by dentists), almost all had resisted surgery, few prescriptions were written for drugs, and most were never treated with antibiotics.

This may exemplify the physician's ability to distinguish those actions and processes that can actually influence the course of illness. As a result, they use modern medicine in ways quite different from those to which the medical profession has been systematically educating the public. Soon physicians will also appreciate the role of exercise and nutrition in maintaining and restoring health. But without public awareness and pressure it is unlikely that the knowledge will be passed on to their patient in a systematic, educational process.

COMMUNITY RESPONSIBILITY

Community responsibility for providing fitness opportunities for older persons is especially appropriate. The predicament of the older population within a community is close and visible to the majority of people in a community. In most cases younger members of a community will themselves become categorized as "seniors." It should also be appreciated that the increased vitality and productivity of older persons can directly benefit the cultural and intellectual development of a community. The talents and wisdom of older people can only be enjoyed if there is health and fitness with which to disperse them.

One organization designed to encourage community support of fitness programs for older Americans is the National Association for Human Development. This nonprofit organization assists the aged in meeting social, physical, economic, and intellectual needs. They are especially concerned about the lack of health education and information emphasizing the importance of physical activity for the elderly. They have information which may be useful to someone interested in developing a community fitness program for senior citizens. Their address is: 1750 Pennsylvania Ave., N.E. Washington, D.C.

Another important community service designed for older people and people with heart disease is "YMCArdiac Therapy." This program is under the auspices of the Nationwide Y.M.C.A. Cardiovascular Health Program and is available in several communities. With appropriate community support it could become available in many more.

YMCArdiac Therapy is intended for all coronary-stricken patients, including those debilitated by myocardiac infarction or prior coronary bypass surgery, as well as for those with only partial or no incapacity. The program is the first exercise-based program for cardiacs specifically designed to lower all cardiac risk factors and to study new ways to do so through participant education and behavior modification. It will provide, for the first time, a network of programs involving an enormous structured population of coronary patients using comparable protocols under common sponsorship, eventually linked by computer, among whom can be studied a variety of techniques for exercise testing, therapy, and education.

Another exercise and health education program designed for individuals with heart disease was developed under the auspices of the American Heart Association and is called "Sharing and Caring." This program organizes groups of eight to twenty-nine participants who meet together in informal surroundings to discuss common needs and apprehensions. Professional consultants work with participants and help dispel fears and medical myths. Group leaders are nurses, social workers, and concerned citizens who all have one common quality:they care and are willing to share their time and knowledge.

"Sharing and Caring" is typically a low-cost program. A ten week session should cost less than two hundred dollars. More information about the program is available from the A.H.A. at 15 Bettswood Rd., Norwalk, CT. 06851.

FAMILY RESPONSIBILITY

As has been noted previously, the children of an older parent are faced with difficult decisions regarding responsibility for the health and well-being of parents growing more and more dependent upon others for survival. The stigma and cost of placing such individuals in nursing homes is just slightly less deplorable than maintaining such people in one's own home. In spite of such frankness, it cannot be debated that an alternative preferable to either would be a fitness program that could help the older person to maintain or regain a degree of health and independence that would make the aforementioned problems non-existent.

American families are often guilty of the same projections associated with medical recommendations for the elderly. Parents are often urged by their adult children to remain inactive. Misperceptions regarding the safety and importance of physical activity are largely responsible for these attitudes, but there are psychological reasons as well. Some individuals sincerely believe that their parents deserve a "rest" in recompense for the many years devoted to child-rearing. Other individuals no longer desire the active participation of their parents in affairs that relate to their own existence. The younger adult sometimes wishes to live his or her own life without any further enthusiastic guidance or assistance from elders. In these cases as well, encouraging inactivity may be seen as a solution.

Such responses illustrate that family responsibility for providing fitness programs for senior citizen members includes a responsibility for total family education in this area. The continuation of family support and love is an important component in the psychological well-being of senior citizens and that support must be aimed in the right direction.

PERSONAL RESPONSIBILITY

It is certainly incorrect to assume that most older people do not have the mental capacities with which to make intelligent decisions regarding their own future. Many older individuals who have read or heard about the benefits of proper exercise and nutrition for seniors have taken it upon themselves to enroll in available fitness classes or cardiac therapy programs. Many have modified their own diets and lifestyle patterns. Many have taken up walking or bicycle riding on a regular basis.

Senior citizens can also form self-help groups for individuals with common physical fitness-related needs. Such programs have been very successful in coping with certain social, physical, and emotional problems. A well-known example is Alcoholics Anonymous. In general, the initiative for forming such groups has been derived from those in need of help, without any participation or encouragement by members of the medical community.

It must be remembered that the ultimate goal of a fitness program for seniors is to allow them to remain in control of their own destiny. Although the majority of older people cannot be expected to provide adequate education, funding, facilities, and leadership for fitness programs, they should be expected to help initiate action toward the development of these components. They should be willing to go before appropriate agencies and request, even demand, that the development of fitness programs for senior citizens be given a high priority.

16

GETTING ON WITH
THE PROGRAM

The need for supervision of an exercise program for older persons may be more critical than supervision of younger populations. This assumption recognizes a linear relationship between aging and increased risk factors for heart attack and injury potential. It should be noted that this relationship is neither automatic nor necessary. Medical supervision will be less crucial for someone aged seventy who has maintained a healthful lifestyle than for someone forty who has not. If both individuals had maintained the same lifestyle, however, the additional accumulation of negative stresses in combination with the reduced capabilities associated with true aging processes would dictate a greater need for supervision of the older individuals.

Proper supervision of an exercise program for seniors must include physiological, psychological, and educational monitoring. Physiological monitoring of exercise refers to electrocardiogram observations, pulse rate and blood pressure observations, and watching for signs of fatigue or angina. As has been noted previously, the use of an ECG exercise test is subject to debate. Considering the increased risks of initiating an exercise program for the elderly, however, it is appropriate to discuss the issue further in this section.

There are four major objectives of an ECG stress test for older persons. They include:

- identification of coronary heart disease
- recommendation as to involvement in an exercise program
- prescription for exercise
- legal protection

The first objective, identification of heart disease, poses a question that relates to the other three. If diagnosis indicates heart disease, an individual has detected the possible origin of a symptom. He or she is then faced with the decision of whether or not to intervene with lifestyle modification and exercise, surgery, or medication. This decision will be largely based upon the physician's recommendation, which in turn will be based on the type of heart disease, the physician's understanding of exercise principles, and his concern over legal liability.

Considering the questionable reliability of ECG interpretation and the fact that the majority of individuals with ischemic and non-ischemic heart disease can benefit from proper exercise, a recommendation not to exercise should elicit serious re-evaluation. Although there are several experimental studies that suggest that exercise may have a harmful effect in certain types of cardiomyopathy, such cases are relatively few.

The following prevalent conditions have been found to benefit from proper physical exercise intervention, according to the American Heart Association's *Physicians Handbook on Exercise Training for Heart Patients*:

1. Coronary Heart Disease
   a. angina pectoris
   b. post-myocardial infarction
   c. post-operative vein bypass patients
   d. inadequate pumping function of the heart following post-ventricular aneurysm resection
2. Non-ischemic Heart Disease
   a. post-repair of congenital defects
   b. post-valve replacement (there is yet no evidence that exercise can improve functional capacity in valvular disease)
   c. hypertensive cardiovascular disease
3. Potential Heart Disease
   a. apparent tachyarrhythmias
   b. sinus tachycardia and hyperkinetic states
   c. chronic lung disease
   d. alcoholism

Proper physical activity and lifestyle intervention may also prevent limitations in physical capacities in individuals with sub-clinical heart disease where there are abnormal ECG tracings without actual symptoms. Since it is possible that the ECG manifestation is merely a false positive and since proper exercise is appropriate for individuals even if the ECG segment is an accurate appraisal, a failure to recommend exercise would again be subject to re-evaluation.

Even where there is no evidence that exercise can improve the functional capacity of the cardiovascular system, as in certain types of valvular and congenital disease, it still stands that exercise can improve an older person's capacity for living in other ways. Unless there is evidence to indicate that proper exercise would complicate the heart problem, improvements in the musculo-skeletal and the nervous system can still increase the quality of an older person's life.

The emphasis on the word "proper" in relation to an exercise program for older persons brings the discussion to the third objective of ECG monitoring, i.e., exercise prescription. Here is where the use of medical monitoring of an exercise test for older persons has its most valid application.

The consensus among fitness experts is that only a maximal exercise test can provide an accurate assessment of an older, sedentary individual. The majority of the members of the American Heart Association's Exercise Committee stated that "extrapolation from the sub-maximal measurement to estimated prediction of maximum performance capacity in cardiac patients or in older, sedentary adults is considered highly unreliable by the majority of this committee."

There are two reasons why knowing actual maximum capacities for older, sedentary people is important. First of all, cardiovascular complications are more likely during work efforts that approach actual maximum capacities. Since maximum capacities are lower in older individuals, it is more likely that they would engage in an activity that would incur a potentially hazardous workload than would a younger individual. If older people know their maximal capacity accurately, various workloads involving both exercise and normal activities can be quantified in terms of a safe percentage of that workload.

The M.E.T. system is often used for such guidelines. Tests have been developed so that various workloads approximate a multiple of the oxygen use at rest. One M.E.T. is equal to 3.5 milliliters of oxygen per kilogram of body weight per minute. Exercise prescriptions are also given in terms of the caloric burning value of activities. The most common, however, is the assigning of a safe training heart rate.

The second reason a maximal test should be used for exercise prescription for older persons is because symptomatic limiting discomforts might be determined at a work intensity greater than that usually reached during a sub-maximal test. In most cases this workload will be less than a maximum physiologic capacity, but for practical purposes the point at which the discomfort was felt should be considered maximum. A safe percentage of this maximum would most likely dictate a training heart rate less than what would have been prescribed using the sub-maximal test.

If the maximal test is the best way to prescribe the safest, most efficient workload, the use of ECG equipment and trained medical personnel is the best way to conduct a maximal test on older, higher risk people. The use of ECG monitoring can augment an understanding of clinical responses. In the absense of a sign or symptom of overstress, an abnormal segment displacement can indicate increased risk of heart attack at that workload. Even if the abnormal response is a false positive, a recommendation for exercise based on a percentage of the heart rate at that workload will usually be satisfactory for improving fitness—even if the added caution is unnecessary.

The successful improvement of an older person's aerobic capacity is sometimes dependent on a more accurate determination of training heart rate than may be possible by using age and resting heart-rate values without ECG monitoring. A consistent training overload during an exercise training program can result in a loss of aerobic capacity accompanied by ECG evidence of myocardial ischemia which may not have been present previously. According to DeVries, when such individuals resume training at a reduced workload, aerobic capacity can increase as much as forty-eight percent.

The fourth reason for using an ECG tolerance test for exercise prescription for older persons has to do with the concern over legal liability. This worry is largely responsible for the counterproductive actions or lack of action taken by many physicians. They are aware of the legal recommendations not to prescribe an exercise training program without first obtaining the results of an exercise tolerance test. Since it is also easier for both the patient and the doctor to assume the "take it easy" posture or the "take a pill" posture, the results are that most seniors or heart patients are discouraged by their doctor from beginning an exercise program.

With the epidemic of malpractice suits, a physician's concern about legal liability might be justified; but only if the physician makes every effort to involve the patient in an exercise stress test and training program, is he giving proper care. Any advice that discourages a tolerance test or a proper exercise program should be considered malpractice.

One solution to the legal liability reaction among physicians is not to involve them with the subject in the first place. The liability will, of course, transfer to the individual or agency that is implementing the fitness program, but a different set of rules can come into play.

There is a growing awareness that a properly trained physical education instructor may be more qualified to supervise a fitness program than many physicians who have not been specifically educated. Such an instructor could implement a supervised fitness program for the majority of ambulatory seniors. In those instances where the instructor deemed it necessary, a specific physician interested and trained in exercise physiology could then be recommended. (See PAR Q and PAR X concept in the Appendix)

If an independent agency or individual were thoroughly trained in the following areas, and exercise supervision reflected this training, it is the author's opinion that in the rare event that a participant suffered complications from the exercise program, the director's actions could be successfully defended in a court of law.

Non-Medical Fitness Supervision; Qualifications and Practices Contributing to Liability Protection during Fitness Program Implementation for Seniors or for Persons at High Risk:

I.   Qualifications

1. Certified Advanced Fitness Specialist from Y.M.C.A., certified Exercise Technician from American College of Sports Medicine, or credentialed Exercise Physiologist from an accredited university

2. Certified in Cardiopulmonary Resuscitation by American Red Cross and American Heart Association

3. Knowledge of signs and symptoms of excessive effort

4. Knowledge of Target Heart Rate estimates and formulas for older persons (see Appendix)

5. Knowledge of orthopedic considerations for older individuals engaged in physical exercise

II. Practices

1. Obtain an "informed consent" for exercise testing and training (see Appendix)

2. For individuals with multiple risk factors and blood pressures of 150/95 or higher, recommend that they undergo a medically supervised exercise tolerance test for prescriptive and diagnostic purposes. For all individuals the informed consent should describe the advantage of taking an ECG stress test, and that the participant voluntarily has chosen to forego the stress test in spite of the possible increased risk, and is willing to begin the exercise program (see example in Appendix)

3. Develop a planned program of action, with which all staff members are familiar, for entry into the emergency medical system

4. Assure that all participants are taught how to take their heart rate prior to admission into the exercise program, and that they know their prescribed target heart rate for optimal and safe improvement

The educational and psychological dimensions of the supervision of a fitness program for seniors are as important as the physiological aspects. For example, if a participant is not properly taught how to take his or her own pulse rate, an exercise intensity that is higher than the predicted safe range is likely to be reached. Even during supervised exercise sessions, it is almost impossible for a single instructor to know that every participant is within the proper target heart range unless the participant's own assessment is accurate. Every older participant in a conditioning program should be taught to take an exercise pulse rate prior to admission to the exercise sessions.

Similarly, participants should know their training heart rate range prior to exercise. They should also understand the significance of the heart rate range and in what part of the range they should be exercising. Without such an understanding, not only is there increased risk during a supervised session, but participants could not be expected to exercise properly on their own. Since the ultimate goal of a fitness program is to encourage self-responsibility for health maintaining activities, the importance of such education regarding exercise, nutrition, and lifestyle becomes obvious.

The motivational aspects of education must also be appreciated by the supervisor. As has been stated previously, information alone is not enough to cause significant changes in habits and attitudes that have taken years to develop. The relationship between health maintenance and restoring activities must be understood in terms of actual experience and logical sequence. Furthermore, it must be understood that the educational process is gradual and cumulative. As the older person experiences the increased vitality of exercise in the short term, the educational process should substantiate the basis for a permanent change in lifestyle.

How much education will be required before all of the desired changes will be initiated by the senior depends largely on the individual's specific background, needs, supportive environment, and personal desire. The credibility of the exercise instructor is also of extreme importance, as is his or her ability to teach. The age of the instructor does not seem to matter so long as there exists a mutual respect between the participant and the instructor. The sincere interest in an older person's health and potentiality by a younger person is often a motivational incentive in itself.

An interest in an older person's living potential must be accompanied by an understanding of the psychological needs of that person. The ability of a supervisor to monitor the older participant psychologically is also very important. Beginning a fitness program in later years may be like starting life anew. Such a prospect can give rise to many apprehensions, considering that the individual may have already established emotional defenses in preperation for the withdrawal from life that is often the plight of the older American.

Readmission into a potentially threatening environment is a challenging objective for a senior citizen. It is challenging in terms of prevailing social attitudes regarding the old and in terms of the older person's own psyche which has been largely influenced by social attitudes. The fitness program director should recognize the tendency of older persons to disengage from society, and its effect on success in the fitness program.

Most importantly, psychological supervision of the fitness program should emphasize positive self-esteem. Older people must believe they are worth the effort of becoming and staying healthy. They must believe that they can rejoin and contribute to society. There must be a reason for improved fitness before a fitness program can be successful. The reason must include both an improved physical relationship with the environment and an increased influence on productivity, whether it encompasses creativity, personal growth, or helping individuals or society in general. Opportunities that provide the basis for this self-image should be an adjunct to every fitness program for senior citizens.

THE PROGRAM

There are many physical fitness programs that could be employed for older persons. None would probably meet the approval of all the experts, and there is no hard scientific data that guarantees any exercise program to be entirely risk-free. It should be pointed out, however, that the only risk-free area in the world may be the graveyard. If the benefits of exercise and diet are to be gained, some risk may be necessary. In any case, the risks to health and happiness are more severe if an individual continues an unhealthy existence.

Properly designed and supervised exercise programs based on endurance activities appear to be a practical substitute for the activities which are a part of the lifestyle of the high-longevity populations of the world. Exercise prescription for older persons is based on the same principles of conditioning that relate to younger populations with one possible exception; a slightly lower intensity is recommended to safely achieve a training effect.

The exercise intensity threshold for sedentary people in the over sixty age bracket appears to be about forty percent of maximum heart rate, as compared with the sixty percent necessary for young individuals. For all but the highly conditioned older persons, vigorous walking which raises heart rates to 110-120 beats per minute for thirty to sixty minutes daily is sufficient stimulus to bring about some improvement in cardiovascular-respiratory function. For older persons, exercise sessions should emphasize longer duration and lower intensity.

Most general exercise principles need to be underscored for older participants. For example, it is especially important that the exercise program emphasize the rhythmic activity of the large leg muscle groups while minimizing high intensity work of the small muscle masses and static or isometric contractions. The relaxation pauses in rhythmic exercise and the lower arterial blood pressure required by the large leg muscles make walking, jogging, running, swimming, and bicycling ideal exercise alternatives, with walking and swimming the most preferred. If properly designed to conform to these considerations, calisthenics can also be very beneficial.

It is also especially important to have older participants stretch properly. Unaccustomed exercise in older people often results in moderate to severe soreness because of an inability to relax fatigued muscles. Static stretching has been used in combination with relaxation response exercise to reduce the pain associated with the continual muscle contractions that cause this soreness after a workout.

Three other considerations that should be underscored include the warm-up, the cooldown, and the post-workout shower. It is essential to the welfare of an older participant's bones, joints, and ligaments that every exercise session begin with exercises designed to gradually increase blood flow and temperature. Generally, no vigorous movements should be made until sweating has already begun.

The need to make a gradual transition from vigorous exercise back to the resting state is just as important as warming up. Abrupt change from vigorous exercise to standing still can be dangerous because of the immediate loss of the auxiliary pumping action of the leg muscles helping to return blood to the heart. About three minutes of walking slowly should follow the workout.

Another precaution has to do with the post-workout shower. In 1970, the Federal Trade Commission warned the elderly to be careful about sauna and steam baths because of adverse effects of rising body temperature, blood pressure, and pulse rates. Since a hot shower also results in opening up the circulation, it is important to delay the post-workout shower until the circulation has returned to the normal resting state. Even then, a warm, not hot, shower is recommended.

A typical supervised exercise session could be conducted in a school gymnasium. The only equipment needed would be individual mats for stretching and floor exercises. The session should start with five minutes of slow walking in a circle around the exercise instructor. This should be followed by ten more minutes of slow walking while doing various stretching and calisthenic movements that will bring the majority of muscles into play. Following this, the target heart rate exercise should commence with walking, jogging, and skipping alternately. The instructor should stop everyone periodically and count a six or ten second interval while the participants determine their exercise pulse rate. Those requiring less intense effort should remain in the inner circle, so they can seem to keep up with their peers who are exercising at higher heart rates and can be more easily observed by the instructor.

Following twenty minutes of target heart rate exercise, everyone should commence a slow walk for about five minutes, until pulse rates are all below 95-100 beats per minute. For the next fifteen minutes yoga-like stretching should be directed. Finally, after the stretching, participants should engage in a relaxation-response technique for about five minutes. This involves directing slow and gradual movements of the legs and arms while participants lie on their backs with both knees in the bent-knee position. All the muscles, from the face to the toes, should be tightened and relaxed in series.

Dr. Robert E. Wear, exercise physiologist at the University of New Hampshire, conducts a program similar to this for people confined to wheelchairs. He has each participant hold a two-foot broomstick in both hands while they do arm swings, body rotations, and other calisthenic-type movements. Whenever possible, leg exercises are also encouraged.

In addition to supervised exercise sessions, older participants in a fitness program should be taught to take advantage of spontaneous opportunities for physical activities. Emptying the trash, mowing the lawn, and walking upstairs instead of taking the elevator should follow a redefinition of what is drudgery and what is activity necessary for fitness maintenance. Recreational activities such as gardening and dancing should also be encouraged.

For those unable to do vigorous outdoor exercise, there are activities that, although not strenuous enough to condition the heart, can do a great deal for the body and spirit. For example, Bonnie

Prudden, aged sixty-five, who heads the Institute for Physical Fitness in Stockbridge, Massachusetts, recommends the "ten-penny trick." Ten pennies are put on the floor. An individual, bending with the knees with the back straight, then picks them up one by one and places them, one by one, on the highest shelf possible. They are then, one by one, placed back on the floor. Gradually the number of pennies can be increased.

Another technique uses a "pet rock" weighing one or two pounds that is kept next to the phone. When someone is on the phone, the rock is held in the free hand and brought over the head and back down to the side, and up and around. On the next call, the other hand can be used.

For exercising muscles in the feet and calves, a towel or a newspaper can be curled up using the toes while sitting in a chair. Heavy books can be used to strengthen arm and shoulder muscles. The back can be strengthened by placing the head against a wall, using a pillow for comfort, and lifting a chair or stool as high as possible. The abdominal muscles can be strengthened by tightening them and "hitting" them moderately with both fists. Hand and wrist strength can be increased by squeezing a piece of foam rubber or a tennis ball. The chest muscles can be strengthened with modified push-ups from a hand and knee position. A vigorous towelling after a bath or shower can also help tone muscles in older persons.

With the knowledge of various special considerations for senior citizen fitness programs, a director can introduce programs in many areas within a community. The potential for life improvement through exercise for older persons exists in nursing homes, hospitals, community centers, churches, health and human service organizations, community clubs and organizations, and Y.M.C.As. With radio and television, the private homes of older persons can provide an exercise facility.

PART FIVE:
FITNESS PROGRAMS
FOR CHILDREN

17

THE CHILDREN

Children are the future consumers, the future workers, and the future leaders of a business or industry. The employee's children are the main objective of his or her wage earning. Fitness programs for children are a logical extension of an employee fitness program as well as an appropriate social responsibility. Furthermore, it should be realized that the current profile of health among American children is not promising.

Instead, America continues to support an educational system that fails its youth and eventually its entire citizenry. Meaningful health education at the elementary school level is virtually non-existent. Health education in most public schools has little to do with those factors most vital to health and fitness. Study after study shows youngsters in our effortless society are victimized by becoming fatter, in poorer physical condition, and more problematical in terms of anxiety, depression, and frustration. The American Medical Association estimates that one-third of all American children are overweight.

In recent years, studies on hypertension in adolescents have shown that most cases could not be traced back to an underlying disease. Instead, the elevated pressure related to lifestyle factors typical of older hypertensives. In Marin County, California, one thousand eight hundred sixty-one high school students were screened for hypertension. Of these, one hundred thirty-three had elevated pressures on the first reading and forty-four were referred to a physician for further follow-up.

As more and more money is spent on bypass valve operations and finding a cancer "virus," more and more children are becoming victims of preventable heart disease and cancers. Autopsies on teen-agers since the Korean War have revealed many cases of atherosclerosis. Predictions about the rate of cancer that will affect children by the year 2000 are frightful. Diabetes, respiratory disease, and alcoholism are not uncommon among children not yet out of high school. Still, smoking among school-age females and drinking among school-age males is increasing.

It has been a source of concern and shame that the United States lags behind a dozen countries of Western Europe and Scandinavia with respect to the control of death and disease of children. It should not be considered a coincidence that, in tests of physical strength, stamina, and flexibility, American boys and girls also fare poorly in comparison to European youngsters. Nor should it be surprising that many American children suffer from poor nutrition. An estimated one-fourth of all American school children go to school without having eaten breakfast. Considering that eighty-five percent of American food advertising on television is for "junk" foods and sugary cereal products, it is probable that those that do eat breakfast are eating a meal lacking in nutrients and filled with sugar and preservatives.

To make matters worse, many schools offer a lunch that is so processed as to be devoid of sufficient nutrients. Without adequate natural vitamin and mineral supplements (when appropriate), fresh and wholesome vegetables and grains, healthful breakfasts, and proper exercise, it is a wonder that children can survive, let alone be attentive in shool.

Attentive in school? Many children are not. Most children progress through school learning nowhere near their potential. Many children in the United States are still functionally illiterate by the time they graduate from high school. Of course, there are many reasons for this, ranging from boring curricula and inadequate teachers to integrated classrooms and stifling home lives. But somewhere within this range, poor nutrition and exercise habits play a significant causal role. More and more studies are finding that classroom restlessness decreases and learning capabilities increase with the addition of proper exercise and nutritional practices.

There are three major reasons for the unhealthy lifestyles of American youth that must be understood before a comprehensive health and fitness program can be implemented successfully. They include:

● non-exemplary role models, especially parents and teachers

- television
- poor health education curriculum

Teachers and Parents

Most educators will agree that teaching by example is a most effective way of transferring principles of behavior to children. With instinctive wisdom, children react to what people do more than to what people teach. This simple observation reveals a major inadequacy in primary health education. How can a parent who smokes cigarettes successfully teach his or her children not to smoke? How can a teacher who is too obese to walk across the playground without becoming out of breath convey the virtues of lifelong exercise? How can parents who regularly partake of alcoholic beverages successfully teach their children not to use drugs?

Another important failing of role model guidance has to do with the end product of lifestyle considerations. In the long term a child will not accept lifestyle recommendations from a person whose own life seems "unsuccessful" or unhappy. Even if a parent or teacher does not obviously contradict principles of fitness, their credibility is diminished if a child can detect a general dissatisfaction with life.

This does not mean that a parent or teacher cannot occasionally display feelings of unhappiness, disappointment, or frustration. Such a lack of reality itself would not be conducive to learning. However, the goal of health education is to promote social, physical, and mental well-being, and if a parent or teacher has fallen short of this goal themselves, a child will challenge the credibility of their recommendations.

Thus it can be seen that the teaching of health education requires a high priority of personal attention to health practices. "Do as I say, not as I do" is not a valid approach to teaching. A teacher or parent must, to a large degree, practice what is being preached. Children in today's society are often confused by the many role models that exist and they will tend to choose the one that seems to work the best. They will listen to the logic of fitness instruction but only if there is evidence that it really "works."

Two Important Digressions

In discussing the influence of role models on children's health, there are two specific areas of concern that can affect not only health education and long-term lifestyle but health in the short term as well. These concerns have to do with environmental exposure to food additives and tobacco smoke.

As the hazards of refined foods, simple sugars, and chemical additives become more apparent, parents and teachers who are concerned about the health of their children and students will need more support from other individuals with whom the children relate. A well-intentioned grandparent or neighbor can destroy the most conscientious efforts of a parent or teacher with a ration of Twinkies or candy. It is difficult enough to offset the influence of food manufacturers, let alone have to contend with negative influences from friends and relatives.

The harmful effects of second hand tobacco smoke must also be appreciated by those with whom children are regularly in contact. The United States Surgeon General, and other medical researchers, has reported that children of parents who smoke have almost twice as much respiratory illness as children from nonsmoking families. In *Annals of Allergy,* B.C. Hilman reports that exposure to tobacco smoke inhibits control of allergies in children and may lead to dangerous allergic reactions. This is significant considering that almost five million children have asthma and ten to twenty percent of all children have some kind of allergy.

A health survey in Detroit by Cameron, Kostin et al. found that even healthy children are particularly susceptible to cigarette smoke. The survey concluded that smokers' children were sick more frequantly than non-smokers' children and that the presence of tobacco smoke in the environment is associated with lessened physical health. Such manifestations of poor health in the short term, combined with the long-term probability of cancer as it relates to repeated inhalation of tobacco smoke, must make people stop the criminal, inhumane practice of smoking in a room when children are present.

Television

A child instinctively and unconsciously searches for a way of life that will provide health, i.e., social, physical, and mental well-being. In view of the many alternatives, children will often gravitate toward practices that most appeal to their imagination and that seem directly related to the "fun" things in life. They will especially gravitate toward these practices if regularly exposed to them. Professional advertisers know this; television is the medium through which they "teach" children to accept certain lifestyle habits and products.

In fact, television may be the major source of lifestyle model education for children. Children in the United States are exposed to thousands of hours of high-pressure advertising promoting fast food chains and "junk food." Toys and games that emphasize cars, planes, guns, and machines tend to de-emphasize physical activity and the human body. Many television programs themselves are subversive of active, stimulating lifestyles. Until values or profit motives begin to embrace a concern for legitimate health education, parents and teachers should place some controls on television for children.

Curriculum

The third major reason for poor fitness among American youth is poor health education curriculum. Current middle and high school courses on health are too often unexciting, uninteresting, and unpopular. The material that is usually presented is superficial and has little relation to matters most vital to children at that age. In the majority of schools, health education is taught by athletic coaches and physical education majors who have little background in lifetime health, fitness, and nutritional matters. Traditional physical education curriculum is actually a misnomer and would be more accurately described as sports or games education.

The competitive sports influence on health education and fitness programs in public schools may be a major reason why so many American adults are not motivated to participate in personal fitness programs after school. Physical education classes usually fail to approach fitness on an intellectual basis, with activities selected to meet the demands put forth in theory. Instead, fitness is equated with maximum performance, and physical training for the majority of students becomes a painful, meaningless, and sometimes embarrassing experience.

The potential for embarrassing children involved in a typical physical education program in school is great. The emphasis on performance in the class combined with the social values that emphasize winning makes heroes out of a few and losers out of many. The majority of children in such a program lose confidence in their physical abilities and become unwilling to explore new areas of physical activity for fear of failure. They will relish opportunities to avoid physical activities until, as adults, they re-enter the world of activity in the role of a spectator.

Even children who have natural abilities as athletes can be turned off to lifetime activities as a result of inadequate physical education. Such children are steered into sports programs involving pressures meant and designed for professional athletes. Children are not prepared for such pressures either physically or mentally. Much concern has been expressed regarding sports programs for children and their relationship to physical injury as well. Certain contact sports may be injurious to developing skeletal structures. Improper supervision, injury diagnosis, and equipment are responsible for many sports injuries in younger children. There is also some evidence that "making weight" in high school wrestling programs is damaging to a child's growth.

Not only are some sports played in such a way that they can be injurious to a youngster physically, but mentally and socially as well. Highly competitive sports have a demoralizing effect at an early age when a child finds out he or she has less skill than others. Dr. Gale Mikles, Chairman of the Department of Health, Physical Education, and Recreation at Michigan State University, points out that competition between children from about five to twelve years of age goes against building friendships, gentleness, sensitivity, and the ability to share and care about others. This may not be the outcome of all competition, but it is often a result of competition in which a child engages without the proper intellectual foundation.

There are numerous reasons why health education programs in public schools have failed to provide this proper intellectual basis. Studies of elementary schools in San Francisco by the author and in New York by Dr. Morton Fine have revealed that a primary basis for deciding what to teach is influenced by teacher competencies, and that the majority of teachers are not competent in the area of health and fitness education. As a result, the majority of those teachers studied spend less than fifty minutes per week teaching health to children. In those classes observed, the health instruction received by the children during this time had little to do with developing an understanding of life-long exercise principles or the hazards of smoking and improper diet.

Another problem indicated by the teachers was the lack of available guidelines for health instruction. The unavailability of current texts and audio-visual materials was rated as a serious deterrent to effective fitness education. They also complained of the relatively low level of positive influence from school nurses and physicians. Furthermore, there was no one to act as a liaison among community agencies, parents, teachers, and supervisors. (Fitness specialists for consultation did not seem to be available.) The lack of involvement of these groups coupled with the lack of content guidelines from the district or state seemed to maintain the low priority that health instruction has.

The low priority of health education is further maintained by the high priority in other curriculum areas. The lack of proficiency in reading and writing skills among children graduating from high schools has put a tremendous amount of pressure on school boards and teachers to emphasize these areas. What they fail to realize is that if children were fitter and healthier they would be better equipped to study and to learn how to read and write.

THE ANSWERS

Encouraging lifetime fitness activities among children should ideally be a mutual effort among business and community leaders, parents, teachers, the medical profession, and the media. The potential for directing young and curious minds into healthful lifestyles with such an approach is great. As Walter Lippmann stated in *The Public Philosophy,* "Human behavior is the most adaptable, educable part of the living world." This is especially true with regard to children. Because children can also be misdirected so easily, it is extremely important that Americans begin to concern themselves about the guidelines for behavior to which children are exposed.

The need for structured fitness programs, special facilities, motivational testing protocols, and new institutional values is relatively minimal in promoting physical fitness and healthful living habits among children. If children are taught the value of fitness soon enough, they will create a lifestyle accordingly. They will not have developed emotional stakes to rationalize adherence to poor health habits. Cultural weeds of ignorance will not yet have crowded out the flowers of wisdom.

The fact that education by itself has an effect in increasing physical activity levels was demonstrated in a research project by Dr. Tom Collingwood. A model educational fitness program was developed that emphasized four skills essential for maintaining an individual exercise regimen. The four skills were self-assessment, goal setting, implementation skills, and program awareness. Program awareness described recognition of four components that included rest, hygiene, diet, and exercise. In spite of the fact that there was no exercise supervision or facilities involved in the educational program, a significant number of participants maintained a physically active lifestyle after a one-year period.

The development of a holistic physical fitness and health education program for children can be focused into the following courses of action. After briefly defining these areas, each will be described in detail.

1. Upgrade all programs of health instruction in elementary and secondary schools.

2. Restructure sports and recreation programs at the elementary and junior high school level.

3. Encourage the positive educational potential of commercial and public television programs and discourage the negative influences.

4. Develop parent-teacher cooperation in providing children with a proper diet and a relatively pollution-free environment.

5. Develop parent and teacher cooperation in establishing a concern over the importance of role modeling.

Health Instruction in Schools

Any concerned individual, whether a parent, a teacher, or a school or government official, can initiate the momentum for upgrading health instruction in public schools. The first step is to document the existing inadequacies. An adequate program should meet the following minimum standards:

1. Thirty minutes of physical education instruction should be provided daily for all kindergarten through twelfth grade students. According to the Michigan State Board of Education *Guidelines for Physical Education,* "less than one hundred fifty minutes of instruction per week, at the elementary level, does not permit most students to acquire the competencies in skill, knowledge, and attitudes which are fundamental to subsequent educational experiences and life roles. At the junior and senior high levels, typically one period per day is necessary to achieve sound educational objectives." It is also noted in the *Guidelines* that health education, band, driver education, and any extracurricular activities such as intramurals, inter-scholastic athletics, ROTC, and recess should not take the place of the physical education instruction!

2. Curriculum should be graded and sequential. There should be some coordinated, cumulative direction beginning in kindergarten with movement exploration and values clarification and continuing through high school with exercise physiology and nutrition.

3. The curriculum itself should emphasize the intellectual basis for lifetime physical activity and proper dietary practices. Physical activity and nutritional awareness should be related to work, leisure, family, friends, and self-potential. Basic principles of aerobic exercise should be understood both in theory and application by the time a child is in the eighth grade. Children should be aware of the heart rate and its significance by the time they are in the second grade.

4. Teachers should be able to demonstrate a degree of knowledge about proper exercise and nutrition. Ideally, they should be exemplary.

Once the inadequacies are documented, the concerned individuals should present the documentation along with a letter requesting that an in-service fitness education program for the teachers be initiated. Most schools have enough autonomy to develop such a program without various approvals from higher state authority.

Most schools have enough funding on hand for consultation services to even pay for someone to develop the in-service program. Often there will be a teacher in the district who has the qualifications to set up such a program. If the proposal is properly handled so as not to discredit the teachers, most teachers will receive the idea with enthusiasm. Many will consider it a great opportunity to learn about fitness for their own sake, let alone for the sake of their students. Once their own competencies in the area of physical fitness have been improved, they will be better prepared to help develop a graded curriculum and begin teaching fitness to their classes.

Curriculum development should be an ongoing, properly designed and organized process. The program should be coordinated by a supervisory level staff member whose sole responsibility would be to direct health and fitness curriculum at the district level. This person should be a fitness specialist with advanced qualifications in health education.

Teacher involvement in curriculum development should be a major consideration once teachers themselves gain an understanding of the fundamental priorities. To help provide an ongoing effort at in-service training for teachers, programs could be developed cooperatively by colleges and universities within the area. All agencies, institutions, and individuals involved in developing performance-based programs for elementary school teacher certification should include competencies in health education.

Since one of the major complaints teachers have with regard to the teaching of proper health and fitness education is the lack of teaching materials, responsibility should be established for an ongoing research and review of available materials. Hopefully, more and more materials will become available. For starters the three books listed under "Children's Fitness" in the "Recommended Reading" Appendix are excellent resources.

If the momentum for implementing an in-service program for the teaching of health and fitness education cannot be started with simple requests and recommendations from concerned individuals to school principals, then a more in-depth approach may be necessary. Such an approach will require an endorsement from various segments of the community such as school nurses, physicians, community health organizations, teacher organizations, and parent organizations. With such endorsements, school boards can be requested to implement the recommendations.

For example, in Oakland, California, the California PTA's multimedia presentation on the need for health education in the public schools motivated the school board to establish a health education requirement for high school graduation. In addition, a Health Task

Team was created, involving parents and teachers, to work on the development of teacher's guides for health education in kindergarten through the twelfth grade. The process has taken almost two years to develop but is now being introduced into the regular curriculum.

Restructuring School Sports

If extracurricular sports are to complement, not contradict, the health and fitness curriculum they will have to be restructured. In order to prevent the social, mental, and physical trauma of highly competitive sports, the American Association for Health, Physical Education and Recreation has proposed the "New Physical Education." This program teaches the child what he or she needs to know about body skills and how to use them both as a child and as an adult. It teaches lifetime sports in which competition can be used in a pleasurable way to maintain health or achieve optimal fitness.

By attaching little importance to the winning/losing aspect of competition throughout school, a larger percentage of children can find enjoyment in the world of activity. By establishing the basis for many "minor successes" in physical challenges, a confidence will be gained that will enable fitness and participation in sports and recreation to be maintained throughout one's life. If this confidence is not given a chance to grow because of the stigma attached to losing or to being "unsuccessful" in comparison to others with more talent or higher skill levels, then fitness activities are not likely to be pursued.

The first precept of the restructuring of traditional organized sports is that everyone will "make the team." Too many middle and junior high school coaches use professional coaches as a model and send home the children who are "not good enough." This practice merely dismisses from the program those who could benefit the most.

From the first grade through the twelfth grade, schools should offer a variety of sports and fitness activities. Children should be allowed to determine their own level of success. It should not be determined by scores and comparative performance standards. If a child attempts a new activity, he should be applauded. If he or she improves in that activity it should be acknowledged without too much applause. The child will know that he or she has improved. Coaches and teachers should be interested in the child's growth in physical activities, but should not display an over-concern that might establish a failure syndrome for other children who may not be progressing as rapidly.

As children progress from movement exploration into sports participation, the major emphasis should still be on acquiring skills. Softball games, volleyball games, basketball games, track events, and other sports should be played with children alternating positions. Several games should be played at once so that audience attention is not drawn to children who may feel self-conscious about their performance. Scores should not be kept during sports prior to the twelfth twelfth grade. If less skilled children significantly stifle the growth potential of others on a team, a policy of rotation can eventually place individuals on teams having similar abilities without creating a sense of failure or embarrassment.

During the twelfth grade, teams can be organized in such a way as to provide those children who so desire an opportunity for competitive involvement. By this time children will have already benefited from low pressure sports throughout their school years. Those children who have developed special skills and abilities, and who want to test them against competitive standards, should have the opportunity to do so in organized sports before they graduate from high school. Then, if they so choose, they will have four years of college sports in which to continue their competitive pursuits.

It is, of course, absurd to believe that children could grow up in the United States without some exposure to the negative aspects of premature competition. Even if scores are not kept, children know which people are the most proficient and talented. Outside school, children will still compete to win. However, if a school sports program follows the guidelines of the "new physical education," the trauma of premature competition can be minimized significantly. Children can learn that there is truth in the adage that it is not whether you win or you lose, but how you play the game that is important. This notion will be supported by the system instead of being contradicted by it.

Better Use of Television

Television could be a powerful educational vehicle for bringing important information and new concepts to young and impressionable minds. According to Robert Rushmore, "The thousands of hours a child spends staring blankly at pointless animated cartoons, stylized westerns, stupid clowns, and superficial foolishness represent a challenge to those who are looking for new means of stimulating interest in matters of educational substance. Indeed, the overexposure of children to high-pressure advertising should be the basis for a demand for 'equal time' to present factual and useful information."

Many public television networks are beginning to show programs of such educational substance. Pressure from supporting audiences could be responsible for the introduction of more programs that apply creative imagination to matters of health and fitness. New characters like those on "Sesame Street" could be developed to exemplify proper exercise and diet lifestyles.

Parents should assume more responsibility in guiding children as to what programs can be watched and how much television can be watched. Some of the criteria that should be used for making the determination are included in the following list:

1. Does the program glorify lifestyles that are conducive to poor health? For example, some soap operas may tend to condone or even encourage family crisis situations. Programs that idolize characters who regularly smoke, drink, or act criminally should be avoided.

2. Is the program sponsored by products that are unhealthy? Many programs for children are sponsored by candy manufacturers that stimulate and brainwash children into being sugar addicts. If the programs themselves have some substance, a parent could turn the television off during such commercials. Or, when such commercials appear, parents could use the opportunity to communicate with their children, play a quick game, wrestle, or in some other way detract their attention from the commercial. In some instances it is a good idea to tell the child that the commercial is promoting an unhealthy untruth. Some children will be prepared for this approach.

3. Does the program stimulate thought or imagination? One of the problems with television is that it teaches children not to think, but to accept action vicariously. This can create an individual who is a spectator instead of one who is a participant. If such programs cannot be eliminated entirely, the amount of time that is allowed for watching such programs should at least be reduced.

Families must learn that the watching of television by all members of the family can be a hazard to everyone's health. The habit of television watching is so addictive that many producers develop new programs based on the "least objectionable" theory. This theory states that a program need only be "unobjectionable" for it to be watched by a sufficient number of people. This is based on the research that shows that if the television is already on a particular station, people are more likely to watch that program than to use the energy to change the station, especially when the other stations have programs of similar quality (or lack of quality).

This theory, in itself, describes the potential health hazard of television for the entire population. It can replace active entertainment. It can replace family interrelationships. It can encourage passiveness and discourage initiative. It can promote poisonous foods and unhealthy habits.

But television is obviously here to stay. It is thus the responsibility of consumers to dictate what should be presented. The profit motive is the driving force that can bring about stimulating, creative programming. The need is clear to develop incentives and capital necessary to modify this powerful cultural force.

Parent-Teacher Cooperation

In 1978, the San Diego County Grand Jury stated that parents must be involved for a program of comprehensive health education in the schools to be effective. After a thorough investigation of the status of health education in its public schools, the Grand Jury published a report containing evidence that parental involvement greatly improves a total school health program. Although this may be an obvious conclusion, too many parents do not fully realize how important is their own influence over the health education of their children. This is especially true of diet and drug abuse education.

If parents who are truly concerned about the health and future of their children are unsure about their own knowledge of health and fitness education, they should be willing to initiate steps with which to begin educating themselves. An understanding of principles in this book and in those books listed in the Appendix may be enough to educate parents. There are also adult education classes and holistic health and fitness seminars within most communities.

Not only will children learn from the lifestyle mandated by parents, they can also suffer directly if those lifestyles are faulty. Although the human body is very durable and can adapt to many stresses, there is no doubt that children exposed to poor nutrition, second-hand tobacco smoke, and continual emotional strife are being seriously impaired. Even if parents cannot control the outside environment into which their children must go, if they can control the home environment it is so much the better. If parents continue to feed children highly processed "convenience" foods, highly sugared snacks and candies, and unbalanced meals, it will be difficult for children to understand or apply information that they may be learning in school about the harm of such practices.

Similarly, if parents continue to smoke and abuse alcohol and other drugs in the presence of their children, the children will suffer the harmful effects as directly as if they were themselves abusing the drugs. With the smoking this may be physiologically direct. With the drug abuse, the effect may result from child abuse or neglect. Regardless of the degree of influence or harm, parents must realize that they can undo the positive influences of school education to a significant degree.

Role Models

Even if parents and teachers manage to teach children the proper principles of healthful lifestyles and provide them with appropriate diets and opportunities for exercise, the learning experience may be incomplete if the child's most influential role models contradict the lessons.

The importance of parent and teacher role modeling should be obvious by now. The solution, however, is challenging. Parents and teachers may feel that they have no responsibility to change their own lifestyle for the sake of their children and students. However, both groups have automatically accepted that responsibility when they chose to be parents or teachers. Individuals who feel no responsibility for setting an example for children have no legitimate right to be parents or teachers.

Those parents and teachers who do appreciate the significance of the educational influence of role modeling have a challenging task ahead of them. But the rewards of changing to a lifestyle that is healthy are not limited to success in teaching children effectively. Adults who quit smoking and begin exercising and watching their diet will benefit from their own increased potential as well as from the satisfaction of having helped the children.

It must be remembered that the ultimate objective of proper health education is to get individuals to take responsibility for their own health. The role of health education is not to mandate healthy lifestyles. Children must learn to use processess of evaluating lifestyles themselves. They must be able to choose from alternatives, make their own compromises, take risks that seem appropriate, and minimize unnecessary habits as best they can. It is not fair, however, to expect the young child to reject alternatives exemplified by those he or she loves and by those with whom he or she is most frequently in contact.

Proper health education should teach children the relationship between health principles and the living world. Life cannot be broken into arbitrary and disconnected hunks of subject matter. How parents and teachers live is as important as what health principles they practice. If physical fitness programs are supposed to make children unafraid to try the difficult, then the directors of health and fitness programs should exemplify a willingness to do the same.

This objective is the nexus between the various sections of this text. It describes the perspective in which organizing health and fitness programs must be viewed.

198

APPENDIX A—TRAINING HEART RATE

The physiological and biochemical changes associated with improving cardiovascular fitness occur when training intensity is between sixty and eighty percent of an individual's aerobic capacity or maximum oxygen intake capability. Research has also shown that sixty to eighty percent of aerobic capacity is equal to seventy to ninety percent of maximum attainable heart rate. Exercising at an intensity above this range will not allow aerobic mechanisms within the body to continue operating. Exercising above this range also presents a higher risk of heart attack in previously sedentary individuals. With few exceptions, exercising at an intensity below this range is not sufficient to bring about desired changes in the cardiovascular system.

Exceptions relate to older persons (over sixty-five and persons recuperating from prolonged bed rest. According to DeVries, significant cardiovascular improvements occured in older populations at as little as fourty percent of aerobic capacity. He recommends a range for older sedentary individuals of fourty to seventy-five percent.

In all cases, beginning exercise programs should recommend a target heart rate range that is in the lower ten percent of the total range for participants during the first six months of the program. Such recommendations should be augmented with recommendations that participants "listen to their bodies" to determine the appropriate heart rate. For example, they should be breathing in large amounts of oxygen but they should not be getting "out of breath." If they cannot carry on a conversation without great difficulty, they are probably exercising at too great an intensity.

An individual has two choices for use of heart rate monitoring that will achieve desired results. The first is to maintain the target heart rate for the entire twenty to fourty-five minute session. The second is to do intervals during which higher intensity exercise is followed by lower intensity exercise in succession. This second alternative is recommended for older individuals. It is important to remember, however, that the heart rate should remain within the range during both cycles of the interval training.

To determine that exercise is being accomplished within the training zone, a participant must learn how to take his or her own pulse (unless a heart rate monitor is being used). Since it is difficult to count a pulse rate during exercise, it must be counted immediately after exercise. Although the pulse rate immediately after exercise is similar to that during exercise, it will begin to drop rapidly. For this reason, the pulse rate should be taken for only six or ten seconds immediately after temporarily stopping the exercise. (To determine beats perminute for a six second count multiply by ten. To determine beats per minute for a ten second count, multiply by six.)

For example, an individual begins running after an adequate warm-up at a comfortable pace. Within a few minutes he stops and feels for a pulse at the radial or carotid artery (at the base of the thumb at the wrist or the notch in the throat next to the adams apple). He immediately counts the number of beats felt in six seconds and resumes running. If the number of beats is above the stipulated training heart rate determined by the formula (below), he will slow down the intensity or speed. If the number of beats per minute is below the stipulated training heart rate, the intensity or speed will be increased accordingly.

To determine the training heart rate, the following formula can be used. The formula is known as the Karvonen formula after the researcher who introduced it. It considers corrent condition via the inclusion of the resting heart rate while standing.

Computing Training Heart Rates

1. Determine maximum attainable heart rate from exercise test or by subtracting your age from 220.
2. Subtract the resting pulse rate (standing position) from the actual or estimated maximum attainable heart rate.
3. Choose appropriate percentage of maximum aerobic capacity as discussed above. For most people, seventy percent will be appropriate.
4. Multiply the percentage number times the remainder found in No. 2 above.
5. To this product add the resting pulse rate. This is your training heart rate at the percentage chosen.

To determine the range, repeat the arithmetic for the low threshold range and the high, maximum range.

Example: for person age 50 with a resting heart rate of 60.

Maximum attainable heart rate (220 - age)	170
minus resting pulse rate	- 60
	110
improvement at 70% (multiply)	x 70
	77
plus resting pulse rate	+ 60
	137

Training Rate at 70% = 137 beats per minute. (Lower range, do same with 60%)

I, _____ ,authorize
to administer and conduct an exercise fitness test designed to determine my physical work capacity. I understand that the following tests will be conducted: (List appropriate tests.) For example:
a. grip strength b. maximum number of sit-ups accomplished in one minute. c. trunk flexion d. cardiovascular fitness as measured by my stepping up and down on a 15¾" bench or my riding a bicycle ergometer, or walking on a treadmill (describe appropriate test.)

The possible advantages of an ECG stress test have been explained to me but I have decided to forego such a test and proceed with the program.

During the performance of the cardiovascular test my heart rate will be monitored and my blood pressure will be measured prior to and at the completion of the test. The test will be discontinued when I reach a predetermined heart rate or time limit, or if I become distressed in any way or develop any abnormal response, whichever of the above comes first. Every effort will be made to conduct the test in such a way as to minimize discomfort and risk. However, I understand that there are potential risks that include transient lightheadedness, fainting, chest discomfort, leg cramps, changes in blood pressure, high heart rates, and extremely rarely, heart attacks. Any signs or symptoms of such risks will be a signal to stop the test. My welfare is protected by the presence of a trained technician.

In agreeing to such evaluations, I waive any legal recourse against the members of _____ from any and all claims resulting from personal injuries sustained or death resulting from these tests. This waiver shall be binding upon my heirs and my personal representatives.

DATE: _____ SUBJECT _____

SIGNATURE

WITNESS _____

INFORMED CONSENT FOR EXERCISE TREATMENT

I,_____, desire to engage voluntarily
in the_____exercise program in order
to improve my personal fitness level.

The activities of the program are designed to place a gradually
increasing work load on the circulation and the muscles and there-
by to improve their function. The reaction of the cardiovascular
system to such activities cannot be predicted with complete accuracy. There is the risk of certain changes occuring during or following
the exercise. These changes include abnormalities of blood pressure
or heart rate, and in rare instances heart attacks. There is also the
possibility of minor over-use injuries, although they will be minimized with proper techniques.

Before starting the program I will be instructed as to the signs and
symptoms of possible risks and will be instructed as to proper exercise intensities.

The advantages of an ECG Stress Test have been explained to me
and I have chosen to: ( ) forego such a test and proceed with the
program OR
( ) undergo such a test before proceeding.

I have read the foregoing and I understand it. Any questions which
have arisen or occurred to me have been answered to my satisfaction.

DATE:_____ SUBJECT_____%____
SIGNATURE
WITNESS_____

APPENDIX C—WEIGHT LOSS PROGRAMS

Fat loss is the most difficult objective of any physical fitness
program. It is also the one for which more consumers are subjected
to fraudulent advice and costly, ineffective services. Millions of
dollars are spent each month on drugs, devices, and diets that comprise what Covert Bailey calls the "Rhythm methods of girth control." Weight is only temporarily lost. In many cases the temporary
loss of weight is accompanied by physical illness caused by the particular regimen.

The reason for the difficulty in achieving effective fat loss has to do with the complexity of the causes of caloric imbalance. There is a multiplicity of chemical, psychological and physical interactions that can produce obesity. Of these the most unfortunate is the inherent number of fat cells in obesity, prevention must begin early in life.

Although there are many reasons for the cause of food intake and a predisposition to caloric imbalance and fat accumulation, in the final analysis fat loss occurs when energy expenditure measured in calories exceeds food intake measured in calories. When the number of calories expended exceeds those ingested by approximately 3500 approximately one pound of fat will have been consumed. To lose one pound per week, a daily deficit of 500 calories is necessary. For adults two pounds of fat per week should be a maximum objective. For children, the maximum objective should be one pound per week.

Many studies have shown that regular aerobic exercise in combination with proper diet is the most effective way to permanently lose excessive fat. Not only will the exercise burn additional calories, but certain metabolic changes occur that augment the burning of fat and the regulatory mechanisms for achieving caloric balance. It is important to note that a scale may not accurately reflect fat loss during such a program because the exercise may be increasing muscle density while fat is being lost. As a result, inches will be lost and percentage of body fat will decrease, but actual weight may not in individuals who are only moderately overfat.

Just as vigorous exercise (training heart rate) is necessary to bring about cardiovascular improvements, it is also necessary to augment fat loss efficiently. Unless large amounts of will power are available for diet control, a person who normally has a difficult time losing fat and keeping it off will need to commit an hour almost daily to an exercise program. This is an average commitment for a person who participates in endurance sports and it is rare that a distance runner, cyclist, or walker is ever overfat. In addition to the exercise it is also difficult to remain fat if food intake is ten to fifteen percent protein, fifteen to twenty percent fat, and sixty-five to seventy-five percent complex carbohydrate with less than two percent of total calories being obtained from simple sugars.

The following two charts have been designed to assist program coordinators and fitness program participants in monitoring their caloric balance.

APPENDIX D–DAILY PROGRESS CHART
FOR EXERCISE AND FAT LOSS

Counting calories is often a time-consuming and impractical hassle. However, once several typical days have been used to calculate caloric output and input, enough education may have been gained to continue the program without actually measuring calories.

To use the following chart, the following information is necessary:
1. You must know the actual calories in each food consumed. This can be accomplished by using a gram scale and the information in Appendix H.
2. You must know the approximate calories required to maintain your current body weight. This can be determined by counting calories for a week during which time no muscle building exercise is engaged in and no change in body weight occurred. The number of calories consumed can then be considered your "metabolic constant" or average daily caloric intake necessary to maintain weight. Another way to determine your average daily metabolic constant is to multiply your body weight by fourteen, fifteen, or sixteen, depending on your metabolic rate and general activity level throughout te day. Use the lower number if is low and the higher if it is high.
3. You must knowthe approximate calories consumed during vigorous activity. The following are suggested by the American heart Association.

walking at three and a half mph = five calories per minute,
                    or cleaning windows or social volleyball
walking at five mph = seven calories per minute,
                    or digging garden, or roller skating
running at six mph = ten calories per minute,
                    or shoveling, or handball (social)
running at ten mph = fifteen calories per minute,
                    or competitive handball or ski touring, etc.

To chart daily progress, simply total daily caloric intake and deduct your metabolic constant and your vigorous physical activity output based on the above ratings. If the remainder is minus or negative then you are losing fat. If it is positive or plus you are gaining. When the total number of minus remainders throughout the month (or week) equal -3500, then you have lost one pound of fat. By visably seeing your progress (or lack of progress) much of the frustration and mystery of why fat is not being reduced can be eliminated.

DATE

Total Caloric Input _____

——————— Subtract metabolic constant _____

Remainder (before exercise) _____

Subtract calories used during vigorous activity - _____

Total Deficit indicated by a minus sign = - _____

OR TOTAL GAIN indicated by a plus sign = + _____

Enter total next to day of the week. Indicate a + or -

Mon _____ Tues _____ Wed _____ Thurs _____ Fri _____ Sat _____ Sun _____

To determine fat loss for the week, subtract total number of + figures from total number of - figures. 3500 = one pound of fat.

To determine fat gain, subtract total number of - figures from total + figures.

APPENDIX E—EQUIPMENT FOR FITNESS ASSESSMENT

0024-001 14-44A Cardio-Exercise Treadmill—Green, 0.7 to 4.2 mph, 0-20% electric elevation, 115 volt, single phase, 60 Hertz

0024-002 14-44B Cardio-Exercise Treadmill—Green, 1.2 to 7 mph, 0-20% electric elevation, 115 volt, single phase, 60 Hertz

0116-002 16-50 Cardio-Exercise Treadmill—Green, 1 - 7 mph, 0-25% electric elevation, 115 volt, single phase, 60 Hertz

0116-001 Ultra-Tred 550 Cardio-Exercise Treadmill—Green, listed under Underwriters Laboratory Medical Equipment Standard No. 544, 1-7 mph, 0-25% electric elevation, 115 volt, single phase, 60 Hertz only

0016-001 18-54 Cardio-Exercise Treadmill—Green, 1-10 mph, 0-10 mph, 0-25% electric elevation, 115 volt, single phase, 60 Hertz

0032-001 14-44J Quinton Health Jogger Treadmill—6 speeds from 1.5 to 7.5 mph, 115 volt, 60 Hertz only

0068-001 Model 856 Store-Away Cycle

0126-001 Model 862 Quinton-Monark Cardio-Exercise Cycle

0144-001 Model 864 Quinton-Monark Weight Ergometer

0140-001 Model 867 Indoor Fitness Cycle

0142-001 Model 868 Quinton-Monark Precision Ergometer

0141-001 Model 872 Sparr Exercise Cycle

0121-001 Pow-R Stroke Rowing Machine

0119-001 Model 650 Heartrate Meter—Battery operated (9 volt), three-lead electrodes, elastic harness (specify S, M, or L)

6327-001 Pulse Respiration Timer

3496-001 Harpenden Skinfold Caliper

7047-001 Handgrip Dynamometer

7384-001 Special Stethoscope

7383-001 Exercise Sphygmomanometer—On castered stand, with 8 foot extendable tubing, complete with adult cuff and bladder

3230-001 Metronome—Electronic, 115 volt, 60 Hertz

3231-001 Metronome—Mechanical

10979-001 Hader Aneroid Sphygmomanometer—(with case)

ABOUT THE AUTHOR

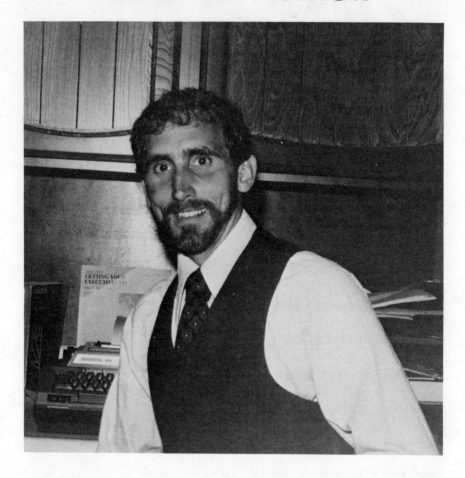

DON T. JACOBS holds a Ph.D. in Health Psychology from Columbia Pacific University and a masters' degree in Physical Education Administration and Health Science. He is fitness consultant to the National Fire Protection Association and a member of the International Academy of Biological Medicine. Dr. Jacobs has worked extensively as a consultant to businesses, schools, police departments, and fire departments in the development of physical fitness programs. He is the author of *Physical Fitness and the Fire Service*, *Physical Fitness and Public Safety*, and *Happy Exercise*, a children's book. Dr. Jacobs is available for fitness consultation and resides in Novato, California.